THE JOYFUL FIGHTER:
A SURVIVOR'S TALE OF TRIUMPH OVER CANCER

JOURNAL EDITION

Jamie Grant-Prater

Caroline Grant

Michael Prater Pharm.D

IN MEMORIAM

Donna Susan Hill
February 25, 1952 – June 29, 2012

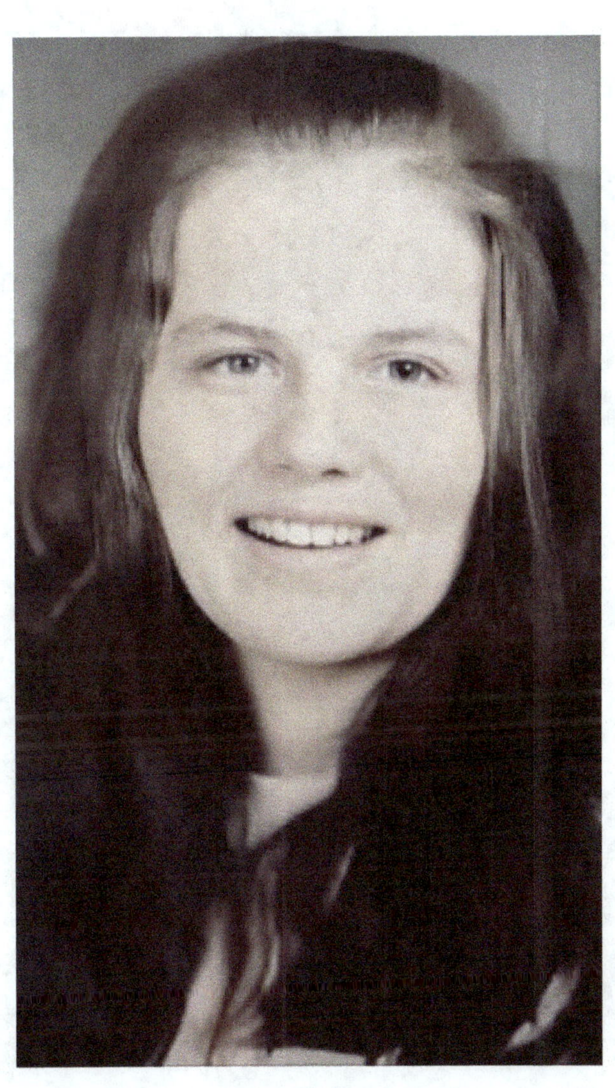

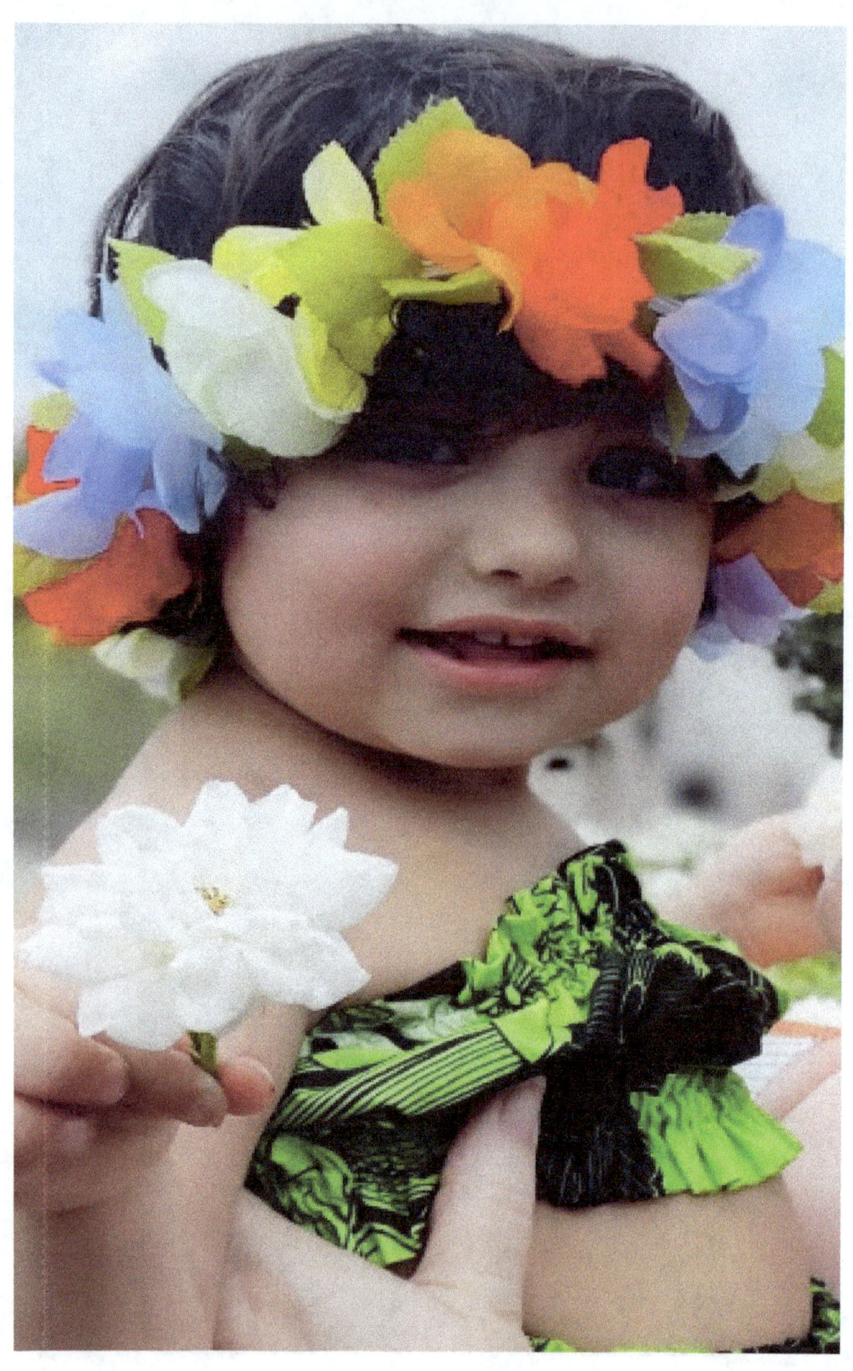

PREFACE

As the sun sets on another beautiful day, I find myself overwhelmed with gratitude. Reflecting upon the journey I've traveled, I am filled with a sense of joy and appreciation for every twist and turn that has led me to this moment. I am thankful for the challenges I've faced, for they have shaped me into a stronger and more resilient individual. Each obstacle has taught me valuable lessons, pushing me to grow and discover the depths of my own potential. I am grateful for the people who have walked alongside me on this path. Their unwavering support, love, and encouragement have been a constant source of inspiration. Thank you to all that have been a source of comfort during my darkest days. Your belief in me has lifted me up when I needed it most, reminding me that I am never alone. I am thankful for the simple pleasures that bring joy to my everyday life. The warmth of a smile, the gentle touch of a loved one, the beauty of nature that surrounds me – these small moments remind me of the abundance and beauty that exists in the world. I am grateful for the opportunities that have come my way – the chance to pursue my many passions, to make a difference, and to leave a positive impact on the lives of others. These opportunities have ignited a fire within me, driving me to reach for the stars and chase my dreams with unwavering determination. And above all, I am thankful for the gift of life itself. Each breath I take is a reminder of the incredible miracle of existence. God is the greatest. I am grateful for the experiences that have shaped me, the memories that have filled my heart, and the endless possibilities that lie ahead. As I embark upon the next chapter of my journey, I carry this gratitude in my heart like a guiding light. I am uplifted by the knowledge that, no matter what lies ahead, I never gave up. I have the strength, the support, and the gratitude to face it with a spirit of hope and resilience. In this epilogue of thankfulness, I choose to embrace the beauty of the present moment and look forward to the future with a heart full of gratitude and joy.

Choose joy always,
Jamie

ACKNOWLEDGMENT

We would like to express our deepest gratitude to Erin Rowland, for driving Jamie to almost every chemotherapy appointment. Not only did she drive Jamie to many appointments, she helped care for our family in every way possible. There simply are not enough words to express our gratitude to her and her family. Her prayers and unwavering support truly played a part in saving Jamie's life. We will cherish our friendship forever.

We would like to thank Pat Prater for physically taking care of Jamie during the worst of her treatment, you are an angel that walks this earth. We would like to thank Nora Hall for holding our family together during the entire year of my treatment.

We would like to thank Karen King-Chadwick for nearly 25 years of priceless friendship. Our children attended the same Montessori preschool and went on to attend the same college in Hawaii.

We would like to thank Georgina Brewer-Kritzer for her abundant prayers for taking Jamie to get healed by Father Fernando Suarez.

We would like to thank Vi Ngo for being the most brilliant, positive influence in our life.

We would like to thank Jyoti Goyal for being a source of eternal positive energy.

We would like to think Irene Perry for her prayers and care for our family during my treatment.

We would like to thank Jill (Sames) Herbold for caring for a young Caroline at Girl Scout events and driving Jamie to appointments.

We would like to thank Tracy Smith for being such a wonderful friend who always made us laugh during my years long treatment plan.

We would like to thank Cassandra and Keoki Crawford for meeting us at the worst time in our life and taking care of all us after my brain surgery. We will love and cherish you both forever.

We would like to thank Anastacia Watson for not only us helping after Jamie's brain surgery but also becoming a lifelong friend. Shine bright always!

We would like to thank Maria D Cecilio Peregrina for being a trusted friend.

We would like to thank Victoria Chau-Vigeant for her eternal beauty and grace.

We would like to thank Cassandra Hess for encouraging us to write this book and our friendship.

We would like to than the entire community of Scripps Ranch.

We would like to thank the entire community of Scripps Health.

Thank you to every single person who ever helped us along the way.

We would like to thank Julie Wright for her kindness and being a bright light during the worst of times.

We would especially like to thank Nicole Beck for the best nurse in the world.

TABLE OF CONTENTS

CHAPTER 1
MY CREATION STORY

At the core of my philosophy lies the profound belief that victory is not measured solely by the absence of scars but rather by accumulating these battle wounds. Each scar tells a story of resilience, a testament to our ability to overcome adversity. I do not speak of scars lightly, for they carry immense weight and significance. This path I find myself on is not one I had ever anticipated or planned for, yet here I stand, fully engaged in a spirited battle, not simply surviving but embracing life with unwavering passion and enthusiasm. I often refer to it as living my beautiful life—a life adorned with scars but filled with triumph and strength.

Now, you may wonder, what is the secret to becoming a joyful warrior amidst the challenges we face? The answer lies in our ability to distinguish between different types of pain. There is the pain that serves as a warning sign, guiding us away from harm and protecting us from further damage. This pain, though uncomfortable, is necessary for our growth and protection. On the other hand, the pain threatens to consume us entirely, seeking to overpower our spirit and extinguish our will. This distinction forms the cornerstone of my message to you as you embark on this journey through the intricate maze that has been my captivating, heartrending, and extraordinary existence.

As you delve into my narrative, I implore you to challenge and reevaluate everything you thought you knew about navigating the challenges of a cancer diagnosis. Let my knowledge and experiences empower you to face your own battles with renewed strength and resilience. Take a moment to reflect on your own journey to classify every ounce of pain you have ever encountered as fuel for survival. Embrace the scars that mark your path, for they are not signs of weakness but symbols of your indomitable spirit and unwavering courage.

In the midst of this exploration, when painful memories resurface and threaten to overwhelm, remember the simple act of drinking a glass of water. It may seem inconsequential, but it serves as a reminder to nourish and hydrate your body and soul. Engage in self-care and personal growth, much like planting seeds in any container and witnessing their transformation into vibrant life. These seeds represent your own potential for development and healing, reminding you that even in the face of adversity, growth and beauty are possible.

So, dear reader, let my words guide you as you traverse life's intricate and sometimes treacherous paths. Let the scars you bear be badges of honor, for they speak of your unwavering spirit and your refusal to be defeated. Embrace the pain that serves as a warning sign, and channel it into the fuel that propels you forward. And amidst it all, remember to drink a glass of water, plant seeds of hope and watch them flourish, for in doing so; you affirm your commitment to living your own beautiful life, one scar at a time.

In those instances, when the weight of a traumatic flashback becomes overwhelmingly unbearable, I highly recommend resorting to the therapeutic remedy of taking an ice-cold shower. The sudden shock of freezing water cascading over your body, leaving you drenched and wrapped in a towel, interrupts the onslaught of distressing memories. At that moment, your innate will to survive will ignite, unleashing a surge of energy that I urge you to learn to harness effectively. This newfound strength will prove to be an invaluable asset on your journey through the challenges of cancer.

But why is this knowledge so crucial? Because mastering the ability to transform negativity into positivity will safeguard your sanity and revolutionize your entire life for the better. Each of us carries burdens that we often keep concealed—hindrances that hinder us from fully healing and recovering from the clutches of cancer. We all possess experiences that possess the power to either build us up or tear us down. My mission is to guide you toward becoming a joyful warrior, instilling within you a deep sense of pride in your personal voyage. Why? Because this profound shift in perspective will ultimately enable you not only to conquer cancer but also to thrive beyond its grasp.

It is important to reiterate a crucial fact: a cure for breast cancer still eludes us. Despite the advancements in medical research and treatment, this unfortunate reality remains unchanged. However, we must not succumb to despair. Instead, let us repeat these empowering words together: "I cannot afford to waste another precious moment of my life on things that bring me pain or sorrow." Redirecting all of your energy towards prioritizing your well-being and maintaining a positive mindset is of utmost importance. Your very survival may depend on it, as it has consistently been a determining factor in my own successful recovery.

So, let us embark on this transformative journey together, shall we? Let us take that vital first step down the intricate path that lies ahead. In order to truly comprehend the wellspring of my strength and unwavering resolve in overcoming my dual primary cancer diagnosis, it is essential to delve into my origins and the formative experiences that have shaped me into who I am today. By understanding my personal history, you will gain valuable insights into the wells of resilience and determination that have propelled me forward. Together, we will navigate the challenges that lie ahead, armed with knowledge, hope, and the unwavering elief that we can triumph over any adversity.

I was born in Cincinnati, Ohio, in 1971, a time that holds a special place in my heart due to its undeniable magic and enchantment. The 1970s, in particular, seemed to exude an air of wonder, and as a young child, I found myself captivated by various elements of that era. Cars, airplanes, playing cards, and even clowns held a deep fascination for me, each contributing to the enchantment surrounding my early life. Little did I know that these seemingly innocent interests would later intersect with the complexities of the world.

Growing up in Norwood, a vibrant suburb of Cincinnati, I was fortunate to be surrounded by bustling manufacturing plants that drove the local economy. General Motors, U.S. Playing Cards, and the imposing B.A.S.F chemical plant were the backbone of the community, offering plentiful job opportunities and fostering a sense of optimism for a prosperous future. In those days, it seemed as though the world was a purer and more wholesome place compared to the multifaceted challenges we face today.

However, the hopeful atmosphere in Norwood was short-lived. Cincinnati was still grappling with the aftermath of the 1968 Avondale riots, which occurred merely three miles from my hometown. The wounds from that tumultuous event were still fresh, and while efforts were being made to heal and reconcile the diverse population, the specter of racial bias persisted throughout my time in Norwood. It is crucial to acknowledge this historical context as it played a significant role in shaping the environment I was raised in—a setting tainted by a blend of paranoid bigotry and the ever-present dangers of chemical exposure.

The issue of chemical poisoning loomed heavily in my childhood memories. My grandfather, a military veteran, was employed at the local chemical plant, which emitted an ominous presence on the outskirts of Norwood. I vividly recall him returning home each day, his entire body drenched in a disconcerting blue hue from head to toe. It was an unsettling sight, and my grandmother, with a stern tone, would warn us to keep our distance until he had thoroughly showered off the chemical residue. This became my earliest and most potent memory of toxic chemical exposure—a haunting reminder of the dangers lurking in our everyday lives.

Regrettably, this initial encounter with chemical toxicity was only the beginning. As I grew older, I became increasingly aware of the prevalence of hazardous substances in our community. The stories of neighbors falling ill or suffering from mysterious ailments became all too common, and the connection to the industrial plants in our vicinity became impossible to ignore. It was a stark realization that our idyllic suburban existence had a dark underbelly that posed significant risks to our health and well-being.

In the subsequent years, the issue of chemical exposure became an inescapable part of our lives in Norwood. The concerns and consequences of working in close proximity to these plants weighed heavily on the minds of families in our community. The pursuit of economic stability had come at a steep price, as the invisible threats posed by toxic substances permeated our daily existence.

My late grandmother, may she rest in peace, possessed a distinctive character. She was known for her frequent use of Valium, chain-smoking, penchant for firearms, germophobia, and tendency to pilfer. From her, I learned numerous life lessons, albeit of the hard-knock variety. Later in life, I would find myself questioned about certain knowledge, and I would chuckle and reply, "My grandmother taught me." However, I conveniently omitted the latter part—she taught me what not to do. Nevertheless, it was a lesson, and I remain grateful for it.

She was the thirteenth child born in Kentucky and endured a childhood marked by abject poverty. Throughout her life, she had a propensity for stealing. As a young child, she would take me window shopping, and if she asked, "Jamie, do you like this dress?" and I responded with a "Yes," the very next day, the dress would magically appear on my bed for me to wear. At that tender age, I was oblivious to what was truly happening until she began attracting unwanted attention from store security. On one occasion, she was apprehended and threatened with arrest for allegedly stealing perfume. She vehemently denied the accusation, asserting that she couldn't have stolen the perfume as the bottle's cap was sitting on her kitchen table. She challenged the security guard to accompany her and verify that she had owned the perfume prior to entering the store that day. The police obliged and escorted her, confirming the truth of her story. She proudly held the perfume cap aloft like a trophy, exclaiming, "How could I steal it if I already own it?" And indeed, she did own it at that moment, having previously pilfered it on a previous shopping trip. Such was life when "shopping" with my grandmother.

My great aunts would often engage in conversations with me, urging me to promise that I would never grow up to become a thief. I wholeheartedly made that promise and, for the most part, have kept it throughout my life. In fact, I have been known to give away the majority of my possessions three times over, as if the act of generosity could rectify past generational karma. If you were to ask me, I would assert that this practice has yielded positive results, which may be one reason I am still alive today.

Life with my grandmother was incredibly difficult. I used to believe she was attempting to exhaust me with strenuous physical tasks. Whether hauling a wheelbarrow back and forth from the nearby train tracks to collect hundreds of pounds of river rocks or mowing her lawn in the scorching summer heat when I was just nine years old, my childhood was characterized by strict discipline and laborious responsibilities. The common thread throughout was her constant animosity towards my mother.

My mother, being the youngest of three siblings, had her own challenges to face. She was married when she became pregnant with me, but the man she was married to was not my biological father. The identity of my true father was deliberately kept a secret—a secret that would remain undisclosed until I reached the age of fifty. Not only was my true identity concealed from me, but an even greater lie deeply impacted my life: the falsehood regarding my race. Due to my dark hair and features, I was labeled as half-Chinese, despite it being far from the truth. The lies persisted, taking on a life of their own. I often jest that I must have been born a liar since lies were all I ever heard. "You are not white! You're Asian... you're Chinese!" These words echoed through my childhood, and the phrase "YOU ARE NOT A HILL!" became their saving grace.

These falsehoods would weave themselves into the fabric of my existence, ultimately enveloping me in a protective quilt. This quilt became a thing of great beauty from seemingly useless threads, shielding me from harm and transforming me into a more remarkable being for the world to witness, like a priceless work of art. The ability to reframe my life into something more positive, I believe, has saved me. I cannot emphasize enough the significance of this skill for my mental well-being, particularly during the most challenging moments of my cancer treatments.

Family. Unfortunately, my family became synonymous with humiliation and harm. This was the unmistakable message conveyed by my grandmother. She would brandish her gun, threatening to shoot anyone who dared to cause me harm. I vividly remember the day she fired a shot through the front door, narrowly missing my step-father by an inch and almost taking his life. Such behavior was normalized in our household. At the tender age of five or six, my grandmother taught me how to clean and load a gun, instructing me to aim for the heart instead of the head and eliminate anyone who threatened me.

Additionally, she told me that if I ever felt endangered, I should inform the person, "My grandmother told me to tell you that she will kill you." Remarkably, those words proved effective when I faced a potential assailant who promptly retreated and never bothered me again. While her protection held a certain power, it would prove inadequate against the humiliations I endured in high school or the abuse I would face from my future stepmother.

Nevertheless, I would later harness the emotional scars from those experiences as a source of strength to overcome cancer. Little did I know that things were about to become far worse than I could have ever imagined. The dream I had would transform into a real-life nightmare, placing me in even greater danger.

My mother's mental illness continued to spiral out of control, leaving me to fend for myself for the most part. I have been independent since the age of five. For the record, I firmly believe that my mother's mental illness was a direct consequence of the same chemical exposure that led to my cancer. Eventually, my mother ended up divorced with three children from three different men. The youngest, my half-brother, was born ten years after me and had autism and cerebral palsy—another consequence likely linked to my mother's exposure to toxic chemicals. Connecting the dots, it becomes evident how environmental toxins have insidiously affected our lives, unbeknownst to us.

Now, I would like to discuss the topic of mental illness. Please note that I am not offering medical advice; I am simply sharing my personal experiences with mental illness, cancer, and abuse. I am the rose that bloomed from poison water, emerging from a crack in the concrete. Sharing my story is crucial to help and inspire others grappling with similar issues. Growing up with a mother who has schizophrenia and other mental health diagnoses is undoubtedly a challenging and intricate journey. Schizophrenia is a chronic mental disorder characterized by delusions, hallucinations, disorganized speech and behavior, and other symptoms that impair a person's clarity of thought and daily functioning. It affects approximately 1% of the global population and poses unique difficulties for children and families. From my own experience, navigating life with a mother who has schizophrenia was an emotional roller coaster rife with challenges.

In all honesty, my childhood memories are filled with instances of my mother conversing with inanimate objects. I learned to adapt and play along at a young age, assuming various roles to satisfy her. One vivid example comes to mind: after days of tirelessly working on a painting project, my mother called me over to evaluate her latest creation. The room was permeated with the strong aroma of oil-based paints and a John Wayne Western movie played in the background. As an artist, my mother always appreciated my admiration.

However, in the midst of explaining her artwork, she abruptly diverted her attention and engaged in a lengthy conversation with the television as if a living being stood before us. Though peculiar, such occurrences had become rather commonplace, steadily increasing in frequency. This incident occurred when we moved to a vast rural ranch in Indiana, spanning 22 acres of ponds and a grand swimming pool.

Seeking tranquility for her artistic pursuits, my mother temporarily leased the property. Amidst this idyllic backdrop, my mother's behavior oscillated between moments of affection and support and times of detachment or paranoia.

During the tender age of 10, I reveled in exploring the ranch, indulging in daily swims. However, it didn't take long for me to notice the regular presence of the owner's adult son at our poolside. He seemed captivated by my swimming routine. Oblivious to it all, my mother continued in her own world, consumed by her thoughts. Fortunately, I confided in my grandmother about this unsettling situation, prompting her to decide that it would be best for me to remain in her care. This experience instilled in me the importance of trusting my instincts.

Each time that man approached me, an undeniable sense of danger surged through me, causing the hairs on the back of my neck to stand on end. My vigilance prevented him from getting too close or laying a hand on me, often leading me to cut my swimming sessions short upon his arrival. Meanwhile, my mother remained oblivious to these events, absorbed in her own pursuits.

Some days, she would stay awake for consecutive 48-hour stretches, engrossed in her painting and adamantly resisting any interruptions. Consequently, I shouldered the responsibility of caring for my siblings and maintaining our home, a daunting task that ultimately fortified my understanding of mental health and resilience.

Growing up with a mother who suffers from schizophrenia posed significant challenges, chiefly due to the unpredictability of her condition. Schizophrenia encompasses a wide spectrum of symptoms that fluctuate in intensity and frequency. In my mother's case, she experienced periods of heightened paranoia, firmly convinced that she was being watched or targeted.

Given her past encounter with a kidnapping attempt and her father's history as a prisoner of war, her apprehension held some validity. During these episodes, she would withdraw from the outside world, often refusing to leave the house or engage with others. As a result, I found myself increasingly isolated. Paradoxically, this isolation later proved instrumental in navigating the prolonged and demanding course of my cancer treatment.

Throughout my childhood, I observed my mother experience frequent and drastic mood swings. She would abruptly transition from happiness and vitality to sadness and withdrawal within a matter of hours. As a young child, it was challenging for me to comprehend the reasons behind these sudden shifts, and knowing how to respond became even more perplexing. However, the initial indication of her deteriorating condition became apparent when she nearly caused fatal harm to my half-sister. I distinctly remember this incident occurring in our shared room when I was around 5 or 6 years old. My mother burst into our space, demanding to know the source of the noise. Both my sister and I denied any involvement, blaming each other as typical young children do. However, on this occasion, she erupted into violence, almost taking my half-sister's life. This marked my earliest memory of my mother's mental decline, as she had never exhibited violent or physically abusive behavior before. In fact, her natural demeanor had always been calm and pleasant, in stark contrast to my grandmother.

Despite my lifelong attempts to reconcile with my half-sister, she remained emotionally and financially abusive toward both me and my children. Consequently, I made the difficult decision to permanently end our relationship, which I have come to accept. This choice came after my cancer treatment, during which I discovered her intentional efforts to harm me. Cancer, in a peculiar way, served as a truth serum in my life, and for that, I am eternally grateful. My diagnosis and treatment shed light on various aspects of my life, providing me with the opportunity to redirect my path. I now find peace with everything that unfolded after my cancer diagnosis, recognizing that it all happened for a reason. Every experience, no matter how challenging, has ultimately forged me into a resilient individual capable of weathering any storm.

In addition to navigating my mother's mental illness, I also confronted the stigma associated with such conditions. Growing up, this proved to be an isolating and humiliating experience. Unfortunately, mental illness continues to be widely misunderstood and stigmatized in numerous communities, preventing families from accessing the necessary support and resources. I vividly remember feeling embarrassed to discuss my mother's illness with my friends, fearing their judgment and potential loss of respect for me. Ironically, a cancer diagnosis can elicit similar emotions. Interestingly, my upbringing, where I had to cope with my mother's mental illness, inadvertently equipped me to face my own life-altering journey with cancer.

Despite the challenges I faced growing up with a mother who has schizophrenia, it has been a profound teacher, instilling in me invaluable lessons of resilience and compassion. Through this experience, I have learned to cultivate patience and understanding towards others, acknowledging that everyone carries their own burdens and obstacles. Additionally, I have come to recognize the significance of self-care and the adoption of coping mechanisms such as exercise, meditation, and therapy.

Moreover, my upbringing with a mother who battles schizophrenia has granted me a unique perspective on mental health and the urgency of advocating for individuals facing mental illness. I firmly believe that it is imperative for those impacted by mental health conditions, both individuals and families, to courageously share their experiences, thereby dismantling the stigma and improving access to care and resources.

By openly discussing and raising awareness about mental health, we can dismantle the stigma surrounding it and enhance access to care for all individuals. This important conversation allows us to create an environment of understanding and support where people feel safe to seek help without fear of judgment or discrimination. When we acknowledge and openly talk about mental health, we normalize the experiences and struggles that many individuals face, promoting empathy and compassion within society.

When I embarked on this project, I dedicated considerable time to introspection, delving deep into the factors that have shaped me into the person I am today. It was a journey of self-discovery as I sought to understand the sources of my strength, determination, and character—qualities that have not only helped me navigate life but also enabled me to confront the simultaneous challenges of Stage 3 Triple Negative Breast Cancer and an Inoperable Brain Tumor. Through this process of self-reflection, I found myself reevaluating my past and relearning everything I thought I knew about the environment in which I grew up. It allowed me to gain a deeper understanding of my own mental health and the importance of addressing it with care and compassion.

The tragic industrial accident known as the BASF Norwood explosion took place on July 19, 1990, at the BASF

Corporation's plant in Norwood, Ohio, United States. This catastrophic incident resulted in the devastating loss of two workers' lives and left over seventy others injured. The consequences of this event were far-reaching, affecting not only the individuals directly involved but also the entire community and industry at large.

The BASF facility in Norwood was primarily focused on chemical manufacturing, producing a wide range of chemicals, including pesticides and herbicides. It was an essential part of the local economy, providing employment opportunities and contributing to the growth of the region. However, the sequence of events leading to the explosion unveiled the inherent risks associated with industrial processes and the urgent need for stringent safety measures.

The incident began when a reactor vessel, which was being used in herbicide production, experienced excessive pressure and ultimately ruptured. This initial explosion triggered a devastating chain reaction, leading to multiple fires and subsequent explosions throughout the entire facility. The impact was not only physical but also psychological, leaving the workers and their families traumatized by the sudden and tragic loss of life, as well as the injuries sustained by many.

The BASF Norwood explosion serves as a stark reminder of the importance of workplace safety and the need for comprehensive regulations to protect the well-being of workers and the surrounding community. It highlights the profound consequences that can arise when safety protocols are not strictly followed or when proper preventive measures are not in place.

The sheer force of the blast was so immense that it inflicted substantial damage to nearby buildings and residences, with its tremors reverberating for miles. Additionally, the explosion released a hazardous cloud of chemicals, including nitric acid, sulfuric acid, and hydrochloric acid, posing a significant health hazard to the surrounding residents and workers.

Swiftly responding to the emergency, local fire departments, police forces, and hazardous materials teams swiftly arrived at the scene, working tirelessly to contain the fires and assess the extent of the damage. The aftermath of the explosion was nothing short of devastating, leaving many of the plant's structures and equipment severely compromised or entirely destroyed.

In the aftermath of the explosion, the community united to extend support to the victims and their families. Local hospitals and medical facilities quickly became overwhelmed with injured workers, prompting authorities to advise residents to remain indoors to avoid exposure to the hazardous chemicals.

A thorough investigation was launched to determine the cause of the explosion, ultimately attributing the catastrophe to a faulty pressure relief valve. The valve, designed to alleviate pressure from the reactor vessel during overpressure situations, malfunctioned, resulting in catastrophic rupture.

The BASF Norwood explosion, which occurred on July 19, 1990, left an indelible mark on Norwood, forever altering the lives of its residents. The impact even reached my mother's house, situated less than a mile away, as evident by the cracked foundation caused by the explosion.

The BASF chemical plant in Norwood, Ohio, encompassed a vast industrial complex that produced an array of chemicals, including herbicides, pesticides, and fungicides. Spanning a sprawling 67-acre site along the Ohio River, the plant stood as one of the largest chemical manufacturing facilities in the United States during that era.

The facility comprised multiple buildings and structures, housing production facilities, storage tanks, laboratories, administrative offices, and employee amenities. It employed hundreds of highly trained professionals, each contributing their expertise to the operations.

Following the explosion, the BASF Corporation faced substantial legal and financial consequences. In addition to providing millions of dollars in compensation to the victims and their families, the company incurred fines from regulatory agencies and implemented stringent safety protocols and procedures to prevent future accidents.

The BASF Norwood explosion of 1990 served as a tragic reminder of the inherent hazards associated with industrial chemical manufacturing. It underscored the imperative need for stringent safety standards and a thorough understanding of the happenings within our communities.

As I continue to chronicle this story, I want to emphasize that my intention behind it is not driven by malice. Rather, it serves as a creative expression of my personal journey, allowing me to reflect on the events that have unfolded in my life. It is essential to recognize that each event occurred exactly as it was meant to happen, shaping me into the person I am today.

At present, I find myself in a unique situation where several significant figures in my life have passed away. My grandmother, mother, biological father, and half-brother have all left this world, leaving my half-sister as my only living relative. However, despite the shared bloodline, I have made the difficult choice to sever ties with her due to her emotionally and financially abusive behavior. It is a decision I did not take lightly, but one that was necessary for my own well-being and growth.

During my challenging battle with cancer, the connection between my half-sister and me deteriorated beyond repair. Instead of supporting each other and holding our parents accountable for their actions, she chose to place blame solely on me for everything wrong in her life. This toxic dynamic became unbearable, hindering my progress toward wellness. In order to create a positive and healthy environment for myself, I made the conscious decision to distance myself from her and seek out individuals who share my values and radiate positivity.

Letting go of toxic relationships is not an easy task, but it is important to recognize that it is permissible and even necessary for our own well-being. Life is too short to excessively worry about things beyond our control, and holding onto negative and harmful connections only perpetuates stress and anxiety, which can have detrimental effects on our health. Through my own experiences, I have learned to promptly transform stress into more positive activities, adopting an upcycling approach.

By focusing on the things I can control and surrounding myself with uplifting influences, I have been able to redirect my energy toward activities and relationships that bring me joy and fulfillment. This shift in mindset has not only improved my overall well-being but has also allowed me to grow and flourish as an individual. I extend the same permission to you, encouraging you to prioritize your own mental and emotional health. Let go of toxic relationships that hold you back, embrace positivity, and transform stress into opportunities for growth and self-improvement. Life is a precious gift, and it is up to us to make the most of it.

What have I learned from this chapter?

CHAPTER 2
EMBRACING LIFE AND PREPARING FOR DEATH

Life is a breathtaking tapestry woven with precious moments, fragile threads of joy, and gentle whispers of love. We embark on this wondrous journey, not knowing when or where it will lead us. Each day presents an opportunity to embrace life, savor its flavors, and cherish its melodies. And yet, amid the beauty and vitality, we cannot ignore the inevitable companion that shadows our footsteps: death.

Death, a concept that both frightens and intrigues us, holds the power to transform our perspective on life.

It serves as a constant reminder, urging us to live fully, embrace every passing second, and find solace in our limited time here. For it is within this transience that we discover the true essence of existence.

In the face of mortality, our hearts awaken to the subtle miracles that unfold around us. We begin to cherish the laughter of loved ones, the warmth of an embrace, and the gentle touch of a fleeting breeze. The mundane moments of everyday life suddenly shimmer with extraordinary significance, as if whispering, "Make every breath count."

Embracing life is not merely about indulging in grand adventures or accumulating material wealth. It lies in the simplicity of a shared smile, the tenderness of a heartfelt apology, and the courage to pursue our dreams unapologetically. It lies in finding purpose amidst the chaos, nurturing relationships, and lending a hand to those in need. It lies in being present, fully immersed in the beauty of the present moment, rather than longing for an elusive future or dwelling in a past that cannot be changed.

Preparing for death is not an act of morbidity but rather an act of wisdom and compassion. It invites us to reflect on our lives, reconcile with our regrets, and seek forgiveness. It compels us to express gratitude for the opportunities we've had, for the lessons learned, and for the love shared. It prompts us to leave behind a legacy that transcends our physical presence, one that will continue to ripple through the lives of others long after we have departed.

Death, when embraced with open hearts, can become a teacher, guiding us toward a life lived with intention and authenticity. It reminds us that time is a finite resource, urging us to prioritize what truly matters. It compels us to let go of trivial worries and focus on what brings us true joy and fulfillment.

Beginning the discussion of my life, the start is as sad as it could be. My mother had been molested by her father, and the knowledge of this led to me being isolated. The sad part was that I was already very much isolated, and the circumstances of my life did not help me get better. He was a notoriously mean drunk, and I only ever laid eyes on him maybe twice in my whole entire life. No doubt, this event of being molested by her father when he was in a drunken rage claiming not to know who she was, affected my mother's mental health immensely. I was always her caretaker and tried to take care of my younger siblings as well. I had zero support. No one. Not one single family member ever came to check on me. It would not have mattered because I could trust no one. Being raised by my Grandmother, I knew I would have to kill anyone who tried to hurt me or my mother ever again.

I had to be stronger, smarter, and faster than those around me at all times, for my upbringing was plagued by relentless peril. It may be difficult to fathom, but the reality was that I never had the guiding presence of a mother or father. As a result, I was forced to cultivate an unwavering sense of self-reliance from an early age, as my very survival hinged upon it.

Growing up in a world of constant danger, I had to become a master of adaptation. I honed my physical strength, knowing that it could be the determining factor between life and death. Every day brought new challenges that required me to push my limits, whether it was climbing treacherous obstacles or engaging in rigorous physical training. I fortified my body through sheer determination, allowing it to withstand the demanding trials that lay before me.

However, strength alone was not enough to navigate the intricate web of hazards that surrounded me. I understood that intelligence was my most potent weapon. I devoured books, seeking knowledge in subjects ranging from survival techniques to psychology and strategy. By expanding my intellectual prowess, I gained the ability to analyze situations swiftly and devise effective plans of action. I learned to recognize patterns, anticipate threats, and find innovative solutions to the problems that presented themselves in my tumultuous existence.

The isolation, humiliation and uncertainty lead to confidence, resilience and strength beyond belief. In nature, diamonds are formed by pressure. I can say the pressure of my upbringing has developed the core of my being so strong that I truly believe it played a key role in my survival against cancer and the inoperable brain tumor.

The correlation between my challenging upbringing and seeking professional help as an adult lies in the profound impact my early experiences had on my life. Despite my relentless self-reliance and resilience, the trials I faced during my upbringing left an indelible mark on my psyche. Now, as an adult navigating the complex terrain of life changes related to cancer, I recognize the need for additional support and guidance.

Seeking professional help is not an admission of weakness or an endorsement of the labels others may impose upon my childhood. It is a testament to my strength and wisdom as I proactively address the emotional and psychological toll that cancer and its associated challenges can bring. By reaching out for assistance, I acknowledge the complexity of my experiences and their potential impact on my well-being.

While some may attempt to label my childhood experiences based on their own preconceived notions or agendas, it is crucial to remember that every individual's journey is unique. It is not their place to define or reduce my experiences to fit a narrow narrative. Instead, I choose to embrace the complexities of my past, recognizing that they have shaped me into the resilient and adaptable person I am today.

I want to make it clear that I don't consider myself to have been abused as a child. Although I faced numerous episodes of neglect and emotional hardships, I hesitate to label it as abuse. Perhaps it's because those actions were never specifically directed at me in an intentional manner. Regardless, the labels themselves hold little significance in my perspective.

Growing up, I witnessed my mother being labeled with various mental illnesses throughout my entire life. This constant labeling made me realize that the names or labels attached to her meant very little. In fact, they often proved to be detrimental to her true health, leading to misdiagnoses when the root cause of her struggles was something physical rather than mental. This firsthand experience has made me cautious about applying labels to myself or others, as I've seen how quickly they can be misconstrued and result in incorrect assessments of one's true health journey.

I offer this careful warning based on my personal observations of my own mother. Labels can be misleading and limiting, overshadowing the full complexity of an individual's well-being. They can lead to narrow interpretations and fail to capture the multifaceted nature of one's experiences. Instead, it is important to approach the intricacies of our psychological and emotional lives with an open mind and a willingness to delve deeper into the unique circumstances that shape us.

I advocate for a more holistic understanding that looks beyond labels. Rather than relying solely on categorizations, we should strive to explore the full spectrum of human experiences and factors that contribute to one's well-being. By doing so, we can avoid the pitfalls of misdiagnosis, avoid stigmatization, and foster a more comprehensive understanding of ourselves and others.

Watching my mother navigate her arduous health journey provided me with an invaluable lesson in becoming an expert in my well-being long before I ever needed to be. Little did I know that the journey I would embark on would be closely intertwined with my mother's experiences and that a brain tumor diagnosis would unexpectedly enter my life.

It was during a casual afternoon spent playing softball with my children that fate took an unexpected turn. As I dashed toward second base, an unfortunate misstep led to a fall, and the impact of hitting my head momentarily caused me to lose consciousness. Concerned for my well-being, my family rushed me to the emergency room, hoping to rule out any serious injuries.

Within the confines of the hospital, a series of tests and a CT scan were conducted in order to assess the extent of the injury. To my relief, the ER doctor shared that there was no sign of a concussion. However, in a startling twist, the Doctor proceeded to ask me if I was aware of the presence of a brain tumor. The words hung in the air, leaving my husband and me dumbfounded. Until that moment, I had never received a diagnosis of a brain tumor, and to hear it spoken aloud was a jolting revelation.

With a mix of confusion and trepidation, the ER doctor referred me to a neurologist while sharing additional details about the tumor. The tumor, he explained, was small but positioned in a challenging location at the center of my left ventricle, nestled deep within my brain. Due to its precarious position, surgical intervention was deemed infeasible. I learned that this tumor had been a silent companion since my birth, its growth gradual and imperceptible. The Doctor further informed me that its presence would likely manifest symptoms in my early forties.

Unfortunately, unusual symptoms began developing with my eyesight, including severe light sensitivity. At first glance, I did not realize that this was connected to the existing brain tumor. I gradually became so painfully sensitive to light that I began wearing dark sunglasses at all times. I would be referred to a neuro-ophthalmologist. At the time, no correlation would be made between my current symptoms and my existing brain tumor. But eventually, the Doctor suspected my symptoms may be related to my existing brain tumor and ordered more in-depth testing. The results would reveal that my brain tumor was growing. It was determined to likely be the cause of my changing vision issues.

I would keep this diagnosis a secret until my physical symptoms would make it impossible to hide any longer. There was simply no time to worry in my busy life. I had recently married my true soulmate, and our love filled every corner of my heart. I was a mother, and despite the challenges, I found immense joy in raising my two wonderful daughters with zero help from their biological father or his family. The strength of our bond carried us through any obstacles we faced.

Not only was I committed to my family, but I was also successful in my professional life. As a nurse, I had the privilege of helping others and making a positive impact on their lives. Additionally, I expanded my horizons by becoming a certified paralegal, using my skills and knowledge to assist in legal matters. Life was a whirlwind of fulfilling responsibilities, pursuing my passions, and engaging in various hobbies and activities that brought me happiness.

In the midst of this fulfilling life, I received the shocking news of a brain tumor diagnosis. Despite the overwhelming emotions that accompanied this revelation, I made a conscious decision to focus on the present moment and embrace the beauty of life. There were no guarantees about the future, and worrying about the implications of the diagnosis would only steal precious time and joy.

Every day was a testament to the resilience of the human spirit. The love I shared with my soulmate and the joy I found in being a mother fueled my determination to carry on. I surrounded myself with supportive friends and family who unknowingly became my pillars of strength during this silent battle. I reveled in the moments spent with my daughters, cherishing their laughter and milestones with even greater intensity.

The challenges I faced as a nurse and a paralegal provided me with a unique perspective on life. I understood the fragility of existence and the importance of living each day to its fullest. While the shadow of the tumor lingered in the depths of my mind, it could not overpower the light that radiated from within me.

Life taught me that true beauty lies in embracing the present moment, even when faced with adversity. It was in this realization that I found solace and strength. I became a source of inspiration for others, silently carrying my burden while spreading love, hope, and kindness to everyone I encountered.

As time went on and my physical symptoms intensified, the secret I guarded so fiercely began to unravel. But by that point, I had already left an indelible mark on the lives I touched. My daughters had witnessed a mother who never let fear overshadow her love, a wife who cherished every second with her soulmate, and a professional who dedicated herself to helping others.

Life was beautiful, and even with the impending storm, I continued to find moments of pure joy and gratitude. I treasured the support of my loved ones and the unwavering strength that emanated from within me. Regardless of the future, I was determined to face it head-on, armed with the lessons and love that guided me through this remarkable journey.

My life was so full, and I attributed the fatigue I experienced to my jam-packed daily schedule. Each day was a whirlwind of responsibilities, commitments, and pursuing my passions. However, as time went on, I couldn't ignore the signs that something was happening to my body beyond the realm of exhaustion.

Simple tasks began to feel arduous, and even the slightest effort left me winded. I found myself gasping for breath after climbing a flight of stairs or walking a short distance. It was a disconcerting feeling like my body was betraying me, and I couldn't control or understand what was going on.

Then came the day when changing the sheets on my bed, something I used to do with joy and ease, became an overwhelming challenge. Unrelenting fatigue washed over me as I pulled the crisp, clean cotton sheets across the mattress. It was as if my body rebelled against the simple act, and I found myself collapsing onto the floor, desperately trying to catch my breath.

Sitting there, leaning against the side of my bed, I couldn't help but wonder if this was the moment when the brain tumor finally revealed its ugly presence in my daily life. The thought was both terrifying and validating. Terrifying because it meant facing the reality of a life-altering diagnosis, and validating because it confirmed that something was truly wrong, that it wasn't just exhaustion or stress.

Recognizing the changes in my body and the concerning symptoms I experienced, I wasted no time in making an appointment to see my physician. Aware of the importance of addressing any health concerns promptly, I sought answers and guidance from a medical professional I trusted.

During my visit, my physician took a thorough approach, ordering a routine blood work panel as well as a battery of tests to investigate potential underlying causes for my symptoms. This comprehensive approach included checking levels of Vitamin D and assessing thyroid function, among other factors that could contribute to fatigue and physical distress.

During our conversation, my physician also inquired about my mental well-being, raising the possibility of depression. I responded honestly, assuring her that I was genuinely happy and not experiencing any signs of depression. This clarification was crucial in ruling out my symptoms' potential underlying psychological cause.

As time passed, I remained committed to maintaining my well-being and took proactive steps to support my health. I firmly believe in the power of nutrition and its impact on the body, including the brain. Understanding that certain vitamins and minerals play a crucial role in brain health and overall well-being, I incorporated a variety of supplements into my daily routine.

B vitamins, in particular, held a special place in my supplement regimen. I was aware of their benefits in supporting brain function and mental well-being. Alongside other essential nutrients that I felt my diet may be lacking, I diligently took these supplements to ensure my body received the nourishment it needed.

I continued this practice over the next ten years while prioritizing a well-balanced diet. While I cannot definitively attribute my sustained happiness and lack of depression solely to these supplements, I firmly believe they played a role in supporting my brain health and overall well-being.

Despite my initial doubts, the blood test results confirmed what I had feared—my Vitamin D levels were still low. Accepting my Doctor's advice, I diligently continued taking the prescribed Vitamin D supplement. Surprisingly, as time went on, I noticed a remarkable improvement in my overall well-being. The persistent fatigue that plagued me for months dissipated, and I gradually regained a renewed sense of energy and vitality.

Before this, I had resigned myself to the notion that my constant exhaustion was a consequence of the brain tumor I grappled with. It seemed almost natural to assume that feeling fatigued had become my new normal. I had become accustomed to pushing through the day, never allowing myself the luxury of dwelling on my tiredness. With a life overshadowed by the demands of medical treatments and the urgency to address my tumor, there simply wasn't any room for fixation on my own well-being.

Life carried on with its usual rhythm until a strange protrusion emerged on the side of my left breast. It appeared suddenly as if a rock with jagged edges had taken up residence beneath my skin overnight. I couldn't recall any significant impact that could have caused it, as there was no visible bruising. Initially, I dismissed it as an unnoticed injury, and my husband shared my confusion, assuming it was nothing more than a mysterious, benign occurrence.

Another week passed, and the enigmatic lump showed no signs of change. Concern began to seep in, and I decided it was time to consult my Doctor. Nervously, I dialed her number and scheduled an appointment, hoping for reassurance or a simple explanation.

When the day arrived, my Doctor greeted me warmly, her demeanor calm and professional. She carefully examined the protrusion, her experienced eyes searching for any clues it might hold. After a thorough evaluation, she offered her initial assessment, suggesting that it could be a common cyst frequently observed in women with dense breasts. The mention of "dense breasts" caught me off guard, as it was the first time I had heard this description of my body.

Curiosity mingled with apprehension as I asked my Doctor to elaborate on this unfamiliar term. With patience and understanding, she explained that breast density refers to the composition of breast tissue, characterized by the ratio of glandular and fibrous tissue to fatty tissue. Women with dense breasts have more glandular and fibrous tissue, making it harder to detect abnormalities on mammograms and potentially increasing the risk of certain breast conditions.

Her words sparked a series of questions in my mind, and my Doctor kindly took the time to address them all. She reassured me that having dense breasts was not uncommon and emphasized the importance of regular breast self-examinations and screenings, such as mammograms or ultrasounds, for early detection of any potential issues. Her guidance and knowledge provided a sense of empowerment, equipping me with the understanding necessary to monitor my own breast health.

With my Doctor's reassurance echoing in my mind, I tried to put my worries aside and trust that the strange lump would eventually dissipate on its own. However, the peace of mind I found in her explanation was short-lived. Merely two weeks later, I dialed her number again, urgently requesting an appointment to reevaluate the protrusion. Its growth had accelerated, causing a surge of concern within me.

Responding promptly to my distress, my Doctor wasted no time in arranging an ultrasound examination. While the results still suggested that it was likely a cyst, my insistence on seeking further clarity prompted her to order a biopsy. I simply couldn't bear the uncertainty any longer. The waiting game had lost its appeal, and I yearned for a definitive answer, hoping that the biopsy would not only provide clarity but also hasten the resolution of the cyst.

Despite my attempt to suppress worry, a flicker of unease ignited within me as I embarked on the biopsy process. Thoughts of breast cancer flitted through my mind, but I swiftly dismissed them, drawing comfort from the fact that no one in my family had ever been afflicted by this disease. Besides, I was far too young to be stricken by such an illness. Having not yet reached the age of 40, I had never undergone a mammogram, as the recommended screenings typically commence at the age of 50.

As I prepared myself for the biopsy, a sense of determination emerged. I refused to let fear consume me, instead focusing on controlling my health. The procedure was relatively swift, though the minutes ticked by slowly, filled with anticipation and trepidation.

I remember the day I went for my core biopsy, uncertain about the mysterious changes occurring in my breast. Though I tried to convince myself that it couldn't possibly be cancer, deep down, a sense of unease lingered. As I lay flat on the examination table, the technician who performed the procedure tried to alleviate my concerns, mentioning that it was likely just a common cyst causing the lump in my left breast.

A core biopsy, I learned, was a medical procedure designed to gather a minuscule sample of tissue from a suspicious area of the body, in this case, my breast lump. Using a specialized needle, the technician carefully extracted the tissue, which would later be examined under a microscope for any signs of disease or abnormality. I experienced mild discomfort throughout the procedure, but it seemed to go without any significant incident.

However, the physical sensations didn't alert me to the grim reality. It was the sudden shift in the technician's demeanor and the expression on her face that sent a shiver down my spine. As I observed her, it became evident that my fears had been realized—I had breast cancer.

As I slowly got dressed, my mind raced with a torrent of thoughts and emotions. The technician, perhaps realizing the weight of the situation, handed me a small black-and-white pamphlet on breast cancer. This simple act spoke volumes; there was no more mention of the previous notion that it might have been a common cyst. The pamphlet became a tangible reminder of the journey I was about to embark upon—a journey filled with uncertainty but also one that held the promise of strength, resilience, and hope.

In that pivotal moment, holding that pamphlet in my hands, the world around me seemed to fade into the background as I absorbed the information within its pages. It provided a glimpse into the realm of breast cancer, discussing its various types, treatment options, and the emotional support available. The pamphlet served as my initial guide, offering insight into the path I was about to tread and encouraging me to seek further information and support to navigate this challenging journey.

From that day forward, my perspective on life underwent a profound transformation. The once-perceived invincibility shattered, replaced by a newfound appreciation for every precious moment. Breast cancer became an unwelcome companion, infiltrating my daily existence with its constant reminders and demanding medical routines. Yet, I resolved to face it head-on, armed with knowledge, resilience, and an unwavering determination to overcome the obstacles that lay ahead.

After leaving the appointment, my mind filled with a mix of emotions; I immediately reached out to my husband, desperate to share the news that had shaken me to the core. As I relayed the devastating information that I had been diagnosed with breast cancer, his voice trembled with disbelief and shock. In a desperate attempt to offer solace, he urged me not to worry until we received the definitive results. It was clear that the gravity of the situation had yet to fully sink in for both of us.

Days passed, and the anticipation grew unbearable. Finally, the call came from my Doctor on a somber Friday evening at 6 pm. As I answered the phone, I could sense the weight in her voice, as if she had been carrying the burden of this news herself. I could detect the traces of tears that had been shed, evidence of the emotional toll this must have also taken on her. With a mixture of trepidation and resignation, she uttered my name, "Jamie, it's cancer."

Her words hung heavy in the air, leaving me momentarily stunned. The reality of the situation began to sink in as she continued, explaining that the cancer was not only present but that it was of a high grade and aggressively spreading. There was no time to waste; immediate action was necessary. The urgency in her voice mirrored the urgency that now coursed through my veins. The battle against this formidable adversary had to begin without delay.

Oddly enough, as I hung up the phone, a surprising wave of calm washed over me. It wasn't fear that gripped me but rather a peculiar sense of partial relief. For months, I had been grappling with the changes in my body, sometimes questioning my sanity. With the confirmation of my diagnosis, I could finally put to rest the haunting doubts and uncertainties that plagued my every waking moment. The validation of my concerns brought a sense of closure, even amidst the turmoil that lay ahead.

It was in February of 2011 that the official diagnosis was delivered: Stage Two Triple Negative Breast Cancer. Pathologically it was described as a high-grade, invasive ductal carcinoma. The words carried an immense weight as if encapsulating the magnitude of the battle I was about to face. The classification served as a guidepost on this journey, delineating the terrain and preparing me for the challenges that lay ahead.

In the face of this formidable foe, I resolved to arm myself with knowledge, resilience, and an unwavering spirit. It was a call to action, beckoning me to become an active participant in my own healing. I sought out reputable resources, connected with support groups, and engaged in conversations with fellow survivors. With each passing day, I learned more about the intricacies of my condition, exploring treatment options and understanding the importance of self-care.

Triple-negative breast cancer (TNBC) is a highly aggressive form of breast cancer that lacks three crucial receptors typically found in breast cancer cells: the estrogen receptor (ER), the progesterone receptor (PR), and the human epidermal growth factor receptor 2 (HER2). This unique characteristic renders TNBC resistant to hormonal therapies and treatments targeting HER2 receptors. Consequently, chemotherapy becomes the primary mode of treatment for this particular subtype. TNBC is more prevalent among younger women and those with BRCA1 gene mutations, presenting unique challenges and considerations for patients.

Upon receiving my diagnosis, I found myself thrust into a whirlwind of medical appointments and treatment plans. The urgency of the situation propelled me to meet with the Head of Oncology without a prior appointment. As the details of my yearlong treatment plan unfolded, it resembled an intricately specific coffee order, each component playing a vital role in my battle against TNBC. The plan entailed receiving three distinct chemotherapy drugs intravenously over 26 weeks. Unlike other cases, my Doctor opted not to order a port for administering the chemotherapy. She expressed vehement opposition to ports, citing concerns about potential infections and the likelihood of interruptions or delays in my IV treatment. Instead, I would undergo unknown surgery, further adding to my journey's uncertainty. After chemotherapy and surgery, radiation therapy was deemed necessary, requiring an additional 8 or 9 weeks of treatment.

In the midst of the flurry of medical jargon and overwhelming treatment options, I found solace in my unwavering commitment to self-expression. True to myself and my love for cosplay, I made a bold decision to don my Wonder Woman outfit for my first chemotherapy session. Being a lifelong fan and admirer of Wonder Woman, I have always felt a deep connection to the character. Her strength, resilience, and determination resonated with my own journey through life. Little did I know that the adversaries I would face would be invisible, silent, and deadly—carcinogenic chemical exposures and the actual invasion of cancer into every aspect of my being.

As I walked into the treatment center wearing my Wonder Woman attire, I did so not just to amuse others or for the sake of nostalgia but to tap into the very essence of what the character represented to me. It was a reminder of the power within me, the strength I possessed to confront the invisible villains lurking within my own body. Cancer may have attempted to steal my sense of self, but at that moment, I reclaimed it with every step I took.

Throughout the arduous course of treatment, I discovered that there was no time to wallow, be lazy, or dwell on worries. Instead, I channeled my energy into embracing the warrior spirit within. The journey was grueling, physically and emotionally, but I drew inspiration from the embodiment of resilience that Wonder Woman epitomized. She taught me that heroes are not defined by their absence of fear but by their ability to face it head-on. I learned to find courage in vulnerability, seek support from loved ones, and rely on my character's strength.

As the days turned into weeks and the weeks into months, the transformative power of the Wonder Woman persona intertwined with my own identity. It became a symbol of hope, not just for myself but for others fighting similar battles. The chemotherapy sessions, surgeries, and radiation treatments tested my endurance, but I remained steadfast in my determination to emerge victorious, just like the superhero I emulated.

In the end, the journey was not defined solely by medical protocols and treatment regimens. It was a narrative of resilience, self-discovery, and the triumph of the human spirit. TNBC may have initially cast a shadow of doubt over my life, but through the embodiment of Wonder Woman, I learned that even the most formidable challenges could be met with unwavering strength and courage. I embraced my inner warrior, fought against the invisible adversaries, and emerged from the battle scarred but victorious. The echoes of Wonder Woman's battle cry resonated within me, reminding me that I, too, possess the power to conquer any obstacle that comes my way.

CHAPTER 3
SAVING A LIFE,
NOT SAVING A BREAST

A Pharmacist's Perspective by
Dr. Michael Prater

It's no surprise that my wife, Jamie's diagnosis of cancer, came as a huge shock to us. The news blindsided us, as there had never been any known instances of breast cancer in her family. It was a sudden and unexpected turn of events that we were simply not prepared for.

As we embarked on the journey of understanding Jamie's diagnosis, we delved into the initial testing and biopsies of the tumor. To our surprise, the results revealed that she had no genetic markers associated with breast cancer. This revelation only added to the confusion and complexity of the situation. We had assumed that genetic predisposition played a significant role, but now we were left grappling with the unknown.

The absence of genetic markers raised a myriad of questions in our minds. How did this happen? Could there be other underlying factors contributing to her cancer? The uncertainty weighed heavily on us as we sought answers from medical professionals and researched extensively to uncover any potential explanations.

In our quest for understanding, we discovered that breast cancer can manifest even in individuals without a family history or genetic predisposition. It was a sobering realization that cancer doesn't discriminate and can affect anyone, regardless of their genetic makeup. This newfound knowledge highlighted the importance of regular check-ups and screenings for early detection, regardless of one's family medical history.

The bad news, of course, was that Jamie's diagnosis revealed she had triple-negative breast cancer. This specific type of breast cancer, characterized by the absence of estrogen, progesterone, and growth factor receptors, posed significant challenges for treatment and displayed a more aggressive behavior compared to other forms of breast cancer.

The triple negative nature of Jamie's cancer presented a unique hurdle in our treatment journey. The absence of these receptors meant that targeted therapies utilizing receptor inhibitors, which have shown promising results in other breast cancer subtypes, were not viable options for her. This realization brought a wave of disappointment and frustration as we recognized that the conventional treatment avenues might not yield the same level of effectiveness.

Furthermore, upon further evaluation, it was discovered that Jamie's cancer had progressed to stage three rather than the initially suspected stage two. The upgraded stage amplified our concerns and emphasized the urgency of devising an aggressive treatment plan to combat the advancing disease. The realization of the advanced stage brought forth a wave of emotions, ranging from fear and apprehension to a deepened resolve to confront the challenge head-on.

As a Doctor of Pharmacy with over 30 years of hospital experience, I have encountered various medical conditions and treatment regimens throughout my career. However, facing the reality of Jamie's situation, I realized that no amount of professional experience could fully prepare us for the arduous journey that lay ahead. The daunting prospect of a treatment regimen spanning approximately 10 months loomed over us, requiring unwavering commitment, resilience, and unwavering support.

Triple-negative breast cancer, as we discovered, constitutes roughly 15% of all breast cancer cases worldwide. This subtype of breast cancer is notorious for its poor prognosis and limited treatment options. The absence of estrogen, progesterone, and growth factor receptors further complicates the situation, as it eliminates the possibility of utilizing receptor inhibitors that have shown efficacy in other breast cancer types.

The knowledge of the limited treatment options associated with triple-negative breast cancer cast a shadow of uncertainty and apprehension over our journey. We realized that we would need to explore alternative strategies beyond the conventional treatment modalities, to maximize Jamie's chances of successful outcomes. This realization fueled our determination to seek out clinical trials, cutting-edge research, and specialists well-versed in tackling this aggressive form of breast cancer.

We were disheartened to receive the news that at the time of Jamie's diagnosis, the prognosis for her breast cancer indicated an 85% chance of not surviving five years. The weight of those statistics pressed heavily upon us, evoking a mixture of fear, sadness, and a sense of urgency to defy the odds.

However, amidst the overwhelming statistics, we found solace in the fact that we were fortunate to be part of an excellent healthcare system. Our journey with Jamie's cancer unfolded within the embrace of a network of dedicated medical providers who were renowned for their expertise, compassion, and commitment to delivering the highest standard of care.

The guidance and support we received from our healthcare team were invaluable. We were surrounded by professionals who specialized in the intricacies of breast cancer treatment, armed with the latest advancements and research. Their knowledge, coupled with their empathetic approach, instilled a sense of confidence in us, assuring us that we were in the best possible hands.

Upon consultation with Jamie's oncologist, a very aggressive treatment plan was outlined, which was considered the gold standard for treating triple-negative breast cancer. The plan entailed undergoing almost six months of chemotherapy prior to surgery, followed by several months of radiation treatments.

The oncologist's emphasis on an aggressive treatment approach highlighted the urgency and severity of Jamie's condition. The aim was not solely focused on preserving her breast but rather on saving her life. This perspective reinforced the understanding that every decision made throughout the treatment process was centered around achieving the best possible outcome for Jamie's overall well-being and long-term survival.

Chemotherapy played a pivotal role in the management of triple-negative breast cancer. Given the absence of estrogen, progesterone, and growth factor receptors, chemotherapy became the primary line of defense against cancer cells. Its purpose was twofold: to eradicate cancer cells throughout the body, even those that may not be visible on imaging, and to halt the progression of any tumors present.

The chemotherapy regimen prescribed for Jamie was designed to aggressively target and destroy cancer cells, with the ultimate goal of achieving remission. It was a challenging and often physically taxing process, as the treatment's side effects could be significant. However, the oncologist and the medical team were prepared to provide the necessary support and manage any adverse effects to ensure Jamie's well-being throughout the treatment journey.

The treatment regimen outlined by Jamie's oncologist followed a well-established protocol recommended by the National Comprehensive Cancer Network (NCCN) for stage two or higher triple-negative breast cancers. This regimen, known as A-C-T, stands for Adriamycin, Cytoxan, and Taxol. It represented a standardized approach that had shown efficacy in treating this aggressive subtype of breast cancer.

Given Jamie's diagnosis of early operable and invasive ductal carcinoma at stages 2-3, her treatment plan involved neoadjuvant chemotherapy. Neoadjuvant chemotherapy is a treatment approach where chemotherapy drugs are administered prior to the surgical extraction of the tumor. This approach aims to shrink the tumor, reduce its extent, and potentially increase the chances of successful surgical removal.

Jamie's neoadjuvant chemotherapy regimen followed the A-C-T protocol. The regimen consisted of Adriamycin (doxorubicin) and Cytoxan (cyclophosphamide), which were administered as separate infusions every 14 days for a total of four treatments. This initial two-month cycle targeted the cancer cells aggressively, working to shrink the tumor and hinder its growth. Following the completion of the initial Adriamycin and Cytoxan regimen, Taxol was administered weekly for 12 weeks. This phase of chemotherapy further targeted any remaining cancer cells, aiming to eliminate them and reduce the risk of recurrence.

Following the completion of chemotherapy, the treatment plan incorporated breast surgery. This step involved the removal of the primary tumor and, in some cases, nearby lymph nodes. The surgical procedure allowed for a thorough evaluation of the tumor's response to chemotherapy and provided critical information regarding the extent of the cancer's progression. The surgical intervention was crucial in determining the next steps in Jamie's treatment journey.

After surgery, the treatment plan included radiation therapy. Radiation aimed to target any remaining cancer cells in the breast or nearby lymph nodes, reducing the risk of recurrence. This localized approach helped to further eradicate any residual cancer cells that may have evaded previous treatments. The duration and intensity of the radiation treatments were tailored to Jamie's specific circumstances, with the goal of maximizing effectiveness while minimizing potential side effects.

The A-C-T chemotherapy regimen, with its specific drugs and treatment schedule, was selected based on extensive research and clinical experience. It had demonstrated efficacy in treating triple-negative breast cancer, including early operable and invasive ductal carcinoma cases like Jamie's. The sequence and timing of the drugs within the regimen were carefully designed to maximize the therapeutic impact while considering potential side effects and tolerability.

The neoadjuvant chemotherapy approach provided several benefits. By administering chemotherapy before surgery, it allowed for the assessment of tumor response and helped determine the effectiveness of the treatment. It also facilitated the potential downstaging of the tumor, making it more amenable to surgical removal. Additionally, neoadjuvant chemotherapy offered an opportunity to address any microscopic cancer cells that might be present beyond the visible tumor, reducing the risk of recurrence.

Indeed, each of the chemotherapy drugs in the A-C-T regimen—Adriamycin (doxorubicin), Cytoxan (cyclophosphamide), and Taxol (paclitaxel)—are potent and can carry significant side effects. To mitigate these potential adverse effects, additional monitoring and treatment measures are implemented throughout the chemotherapy process.

During each chemotherapy session, additional medications are administered to prevent allergic reactions and manage side effects such as nausea and vomiting. Preemptive medications, such as antihistamines and corticosteroids, may be given to minimize the risk of allergic reactions to chemotherapy drugs. Antiemetic medications are typically provided to help alleviate or prevent chemotherapy-induced nausea and vomiting, which are common side effects.

Between each chemotherapy session, regular lab work is conducted to monitor potential toxicities that can arise from the chemotherapy drugs. These lab tests assess various aspects of the body's functioning, including blood cell counts, liver and kidney function, and markers of organ toxicity. Monitoring these parameters allows the healthcare team to detect any signs of drug-related toxicities promptly and take appropriate measures to mitigate them.

In addition to medication and laboratory monitoring, patients undergoing chemotherapy are closely monitored for potential side effects and adverse reactions during and after each session. This monitoring involves assessing vital signs, evaluating physical and psychological well-being, and addressing any concerns or symptoms experienced by the patient.

During Jamie's chemotherapy journey, she encountered significant complications that underscored the potential risks associated with these potent treatments. One of the chemotherapy drugs she received, Adriamycin, is known for its serious cardiovascular side effects. Unfortunately, Jamie experienced a cardiac issue, resulting in heart failure, a known complication of Adriamycin. This complication was severe enough to require her hospitalization for congestive heart failure.

Despite the setback, Jamie's resilience and determination shone through, and she persevered without missing her subsequent chemotherapy treatments. However, the impact of the chemotherapy on her cardiovascular system persisted, and she continues to experience residual cardiac damage to this day. The combination of chemotherapy and radiation treatments, although crucial in her fight against cancer, has left lasting effects on her heart.

As Jamie's chemotherapy treatments progressed, she reached a point where Taxol (paclitaxel) was introduced into her regimen. However, her first treatment with Taxol brought about unforeseen complications. She developed a fever, and her white blood cell count became significantly elevated, necessitating hospitalization once again. The cause of her symptoms was determined to be diverticulitis, an inflammation and infection of the gastrointestinal system. This condition was precipitated by the Taxol treatment, and, unbeknownst to Jamie, she had underlying diverticulosis, which was exacerbated by the chemotherapy.

These unexpected complications served as a stark reminder of the complexity and potential risks associated with chemotherapy. The powerful nature of these drugs can impact various systems in the body, giving rise to unforeseen challenges and adverse reactions. Jamie's experience highlighted the importance of close monitoring, prompt intervention, and personalized care throughout the treatment process.

The complications Jamie faced underscored the need for a multidisciplinary approach to her care. Her medical team, comprising oncologists, cardiologists, and other specialists, collaborated closely to manage and address chemotherapy-related complications. This collaborative effort ensured that her treatment plan was adjusted to minimize further risks and optimize her overall well-being.

During Jamie's treatment with Taxol, an unexpected challenge arose—a worldwide shortage of the drug. Taxol, derived from the bark of specific tree species found in the Pacific Northwest and Europe, was a crucial component of Jamie's chemotherapy regimen. However, the unforeseen scarcity of Taxol threatened to disrupt her treatment plan and potentially jeopardize her progress.

The shortage of Taxol was an unanticipated occurrence that could have had devastating consequences. However, we were fortunate to be part of a healthcare system that managed to maintain a supply of Taxol, albeit one that was just adequate enough to treat patients currently undergoing chemotherapy. This fortunate circumstance ensured that Jamie's treatment continued without interruption, mitigating the potential negative impact of the drug shortage on her progress.

One of the common and serious side effects of chemotherapy, including Taxol, is neutropenia. Neutropenia is a reduction in the number of white blood cells, which are crucial for fighting off infections. Given the importance of these cells for maintaining a healthy immune system, neutropenia can pose significant risks.

Fortunately, Jamie was able to continue her chemotherapy treatments without experiencing any serious blood abnormalities, including severe neutropenia. This positive outcome allowed her to navigate her treatment course without the additional challenge of compromised immunity, which could have increased the risk of infections and their associated complications.

However, the use of Taxol does come with its own set of known side effects, including neurologic complications. Peripheral neuropathy, characterized by neuropathic pain in the peripheral nerves, is a recognized side effect of Taxol treatment, particularly when used for shorter durations.

The impact of peripheral neuropathy, as a result of chemotherapy, has left a lasting effect on Jamie's life. As time has passed, she can attest to the persistence of these neuropathies, which continue to be a reminder of the challenges she faced during her treatment journey.

After enduring six intense months of chemotherapy, a pivotal moment arrived when it was time to take a break from chemotherapy and proceed with surgery. Remarkably, the fortunes of life smiled upon Jamie as her tumor had decreased in size, rendering it more amenable to breast-conserving surgery. With the successful removal of the tumor and associated axillary lymph node, a significant milestone was reached.

The completion of surgery marked a significant pause in the treatment process, providing an opportunity to regroup and prepare for the next phase: radiation therapy. Over the course of two months, Jamie underwent radiation treatments targeting the tumor site. This rigorous schedule involved radiation sessions five days a week, Monday through Friday, for a total of nine weeks. With the support of friends and family, she successfully completed all 45 radiation treatments, culminating on December 31.

The radiation treatments, though demanding, were a vital component of the comprehensive treatment plan. With determination and perseverance, Jamie braved the physical toll, enduring the scars and burns that came with the treatment. The end of the year marked a significant milestone—the cancer was gone. The dawn of the new year held the promise of a fresh start and a future free from the grip of cancer.

As I write this narrative 12 years later, in 2023, I am delighted to share that Jamie remains cancer-free. The mammograms and other scans conducted throughout the past 12 years have consistently shown no evidence of cancer recurrence. Her life was indeed saved, fulfilling the promise made by her Doctor.

Jamie's journey stands as a testament to the power of perseverance, the unwavering support of loved ones, and the remarkable advancements in medical science. Through the trials and tribulations of her treatment, she emerged triumphant, defying the odds and embracing a new chapter of life, free from the burden of cancer.

CHAPTER 4

A DAUGHTER'S PERSPECTIVE

A Daughter's Perspective by Caroline Grant

During my freshman year in high school, my world was shaken when my mother received the devastating news of her cancer diagnosis. The memories of my carefree childhood became foggy, but certain moments stand out like vivid brushstrokes on a canvas. The news struck us like a lightning bolt on a clear day. Cancer was never something we anticipated on my mother's side of the family. I had known about my grandmother's courageous battle with breast cancer on my father's side, but I had never considered the possibility of it affecting my mom.

The day the diagnosis was delivered is etched into my memory like a painful scar. We were all shocked, our family trying to process the gravity of the situation. I was scared for my mom, but my teenage mind struggled to comprehend the magnitude of what she was facing. The word "cancer" felt like a monster lurking in the shadows, waiting to pounce on our happy life.

In the beginning, my mom tried to protect me from the harsh reality of her battle. She didn't want me to witness the painful chemo sessions or the terrifying medical procedures she had to endure. But even from afar, I could see the toll the treatments were taking on her. The nights she came home, her frail figure and exhaustion spoke louder than any words could.

One of the most heart-wrenching moments was watching her beautiful hair fall out. It started slowly, strands left on her pillow like teardrops. Eventually, she had to face reality and shave her head. I remember feeling a mixture of sadness and pride as she bravely faced this change. Despite her efforts to remain positive, her eyes betrayed the fear and despair she felt. She tried to put on a brave face, but I saw through it. I couldn't bear to see her in pain, but I also couldn't bear to bring it up and add to her burden.

In those challenging times, I found solace in reassuring her that she was the strongest and bravest person I had ever known. I wanted her to know that I believed in her unwavering strength, even when she may have doubted it herself. I hoped my words could be a balm to her wounded spirit, even if it was just for a moment.

The experience of witnessing my mother's battle with cancer had a profound impact on how I perceived my parents. Like most children, I had placed them on a pedestal, seeing them as invincible heroes capable of anything. However, this journey taught me the harsh reality that they, too, were vulnerable and human.

My mom, once my superhero and miracle worker, remained my hero, but in a more realistic light. The emotional and physical toll of her numerous treatments exposed the fragility of her human spirit. I remember hearing her cry in her room during her second round of chemo, wishing for relief from the pain and suffering. Those moments shattered my illusions of her invincibility.

During one heartbreaking moment, I had to beg her not to give up, knowing that her struggle was unbearable. My plea might have seemed selfish, but I was just a young teenager grappling with the terrifying prospect of losing the person I loved the most. I felt helpless and unable to provide anything more than emotional and moral support.

Despite the pain it caused me, I refused to leave her side. I became her unwavering rock, offering whatever support I could muster. As a teenager, my resources were limited, but my determination to be there for her was boundless. I tried my best to be her pillar of strength, hoping that my presence and encouragement would somehow ease her suffering.

Throughout her journey, I witnessed the transformation of our relationship. It was no longer just a parent-child dynamic but a deep bond between two individuals facing adversity together. Our roles shifted, and I learned the true meaning of empathy and compassion. The experience taught me to see my parents as vulnerable beings, subject to the same struggles and fears as any human being.

This profound encounter with my mother's vulnerability and resilience further solidified my commitment to understanding the human brain and its complexities. I became more intrigued by the idea of EEG analysis and neuroscience, eager to uncover the secrets of the mind and how it copes with trauma and pain.

The challenges of those days were immense, but they paved the way for my personal growth and evolution. The lessons learned during my mother's battle with cancer extended far beyond the realm of illness; they taught me about the strength of the human spirit and the profound love that binds families together.

Amidst the turmoil of my home life, the once smooth path of my academic journey started to twist and turn, leading me down a labyrinth of challenges and emotions. Ever since junior high, I had grappled with my grades, but high school was an entirely different struggle altogether. The burden of my mother's illness weighed heavily on my mind, creating a cloud of uncertainty and distraction that made focusing on my studies increasingly difficult.

In my heart, I knew that my mother's condition demanded my attention and care, but at the same time, I yearned to excel in my studies. This internal conflict constantly tore at me, leaving me feeling like I was constantly failing on both fronts. Whether it was my mother's illness or some other undiagnosed issue, the root cause of my declining grades remained a mystery, adding to the complexity of the situation.

As days turned into weeks and weeks into months, I found it increasingly hard to prioritize school over spending time with my mom. Every moment with her was precious, and I couldn't bear the thought of missing out on those invaluable moments. This intense emotional bond with my mother tugged at my heartstrings, leading me to question the very purpose of my academic pursuits. It felt like every second I spent on my studies was time taken away from her, deepening the internal struggle.

I must admit, there were moments when I thought about seeking help from teachers or counselors. I understood that their support could potentially alleviate some of the academic pressures I faced. However, the guilt that overwhelmed me each time I considered reaching out hindered any action on my part. The weight of adding more stress to my mother's life, coupled with my desire to handle everything independently, paralyzed me from seeking the help that I knew, deep down, was necessary.

In retrospect, I can see that my hyper-independence started to develop during this tumultuous time. It became a coping mechanism, a way for me to maintain some semblance of control amid the chaos. I was determined to carry the weight of my family's struggles on my own shoulders, believing that I had to be strong for everyone. Little did I know that this unyielding self-reliance would become both a strength and a weakness in my life.

The emotions swirling within me were complex and overwhelming, like an intricate dance of conflicting feelings. On the one hand, there was a deep sense of love and concern for my mother. I wanted to be there for her, to offer comfort and support during her difficult times. Witnessing her suffer filled me with a pang of indescribable sadness, and I wished there was more I could do to ease her pain.

On the other hand, I couldn't help but feel frustration and disappointment in myself for my academic struggles. I had always been a diligent student, and seeing my grades plummet was a bitter pill to swallow. I questioned my abilities, wondering if I was capable of rising above the challenges I faced. The pressure to succeed academically clashed with the need to be present for my mother, and I felt torn between these two worlds.

The impact of my mother's illness on my life was profound, and while I certainly wish she had never been ill in the first place, I have no regrets about how we handled the diagnosis. It was a devastating change that shook the very foundations of our lives, but looking back, I wouldn't change a thing. My mother's health was of the utmost importance, and we did everything in our power to support her through those difficult times.

The journey of navigating a loved one's illness is never easy. It throws one into a whirlwind of emotions, challenges, and uncertainties. As the illness took its toll on my mother's health, it unavoidably seeped into every aspect of our lives, including my academic performance. While I struggled in school during that period, I refuse to hold my mother accountable for any negative impacts her diagnosis may have had on my education.

Empathy played a crucial role in shaping my perspective during this trying time. It was vital for me to understand that illness is never asked for, and my mother certainly did not choose to be unwell. It was an unfortunate circumstance that life presented to us, and we had to navigate through it the best way we knew how. Blaming or resenting my mother for the challenges I faced in school would be unfair and unkind.

In times of hardship, it is essential to remember that everyone is fighting their own battles, and we cannot fully comprehend the weight of someone else's struggles. My mother, in her battle with illness, needed my love, support, and understanding more than ever. And while it was difficult to balance my responsibilities as a student and a caregiver, I knew that my presence and empathy meant the world to her.

Moreover, empathy extended beyond just understanding my mother's situation; it also entailed recognizing and accepting my own emotions and vulnerabilities. It was okay to feel overwhelmed, sad, or even frustrated by the circumstances. Through embracing my emotions, I learned to be more compassionate with myself, understanding that it was okay not to have all the answers and to reach out for help when needed.

In the midst of all the challenges, our family found solace and strength in coming together as a support system. We became a tightly-knit unit, supporting one another through the highs and lows of my mother's illness. This experience brought a newfound depth to our relationships, teaching us the value of empathy, patience, and understanding.

Reflecting on this chapter in my life, I realize that empathy is a fundamental pillar in navigating any difficulty. It is the ability to put ourselves in someone else's shoes, to see the world through their eyes, and to offer genuine support and care. Empathy not only helped us weather the storm of illness but also fostered a sense of unity and love within our family.

In times of adversity, it's easy to feel isolated and overwhelmed, but empathy bridges that gap, reminding us that we are not alone in our struggles. It encourages open communication and vulnerability, creating an environment where we can share our burdens and find comfort in each other.

To anyone facing a similar situation, I urge you to remember that empathy is a powerful tool. It is not only about understanding the struggles of others but also about being kind to ourselves. As we face challenges, we must be gentle with ourselves, acknowledging that life is unpredictable and that it's okay to feel lost at times.

Empathy also extends beyond our immediate circles. In our fast-paced and interconnected world, we encounter countless individuals battling their own battles. A simple act of empathy, a kind word, or a helping hand can make a world of difference to someone in need.

Furthermore, it is essential to break the stigma surrounding illness and mental health. Too often, individuals facing health challenges are burdened with feelings of shame or inadequacy. By fostering empathy and understanding, we can create a more compassionate society where people feel supported and accepted no matter their circumstances.

In conclusion, the impact of my mother's illness on my life was a profound journey of self-discovery, empathy, and growth. I don't regret any part of it, as it shaped me into the person I am today. Illness is a reality that we must all face at some point, either personally or through our loved ones. And in these moments, empathy becomes an invaluable companion, guiding us through the darkest of times and reminding us that we are not alone in our struggles.

Let us all strive to be more empathetic, both towards others and ourselves. Together, we can create a world that embraces vulnerability, compassion, and understanding, a world where we lift each other up and support one another on this unpredictable journey called life.

What have I learned from this chapter?

CHAPTER 5
TOO MEAN TO DIE

Hello there, I'm here with you, ready to continue this journey through my life's story. I've already shared some important parts of my upbringing, my belief in life's greater plan, and the inevitable highs and lows we all experience. Now, let's delve further into the chapter of my life where health challenges became a significant part of my story.

My health struggles were undoubtedly the most challenging phase I had to endure. It's a vivid reminder that our bodies have a language of their own, and it's crucial to pay attention. Back then, my health issues crept into my life with an almost surreal swiftness. I appeared to be the picture of perfect health, and even my blood work confirmed it. However, appearances can be deceiving. I vividly remember the day when my once-beloved chore of refreshing my bed with clean linens turned into a stark reminder of my vulnerability. You see, I had this passion for turning my bedroom into a sanctuary that mirrored the comforts of a luxury hotel. The aroma and crispness of freshly laundered cotton sheets were like a therapeutic indulgence. It was something I looked forward to every week, a simple pleasure.

But on one fateful afternoon during my usual bed-making ritual, something felt off. As I gently smoothed out the fresh sheets, I felt an unusual tightness in my chest, and a deep fatigue washed over me. It was as though an invisible weight had settled upon my shoulders, making it increasingly difficult to breathe. I lowered myself to the floor, next to my freshly made bed, and that's when it really hit me – I couldn't easily stand back up. The physical and emotional exhaustion overwhelmed me. This fatigue became an unwelcome companion in my daily life. Every task, no matter how simple, felt like a Herculean effort. I knew deep down that something was terribly wrong with my body, but I tried to convince myself it was just a side effect of my preexisting brain tumor diagnosis. This, my friends, is where my story takes an important turn, one filled with cautionary lessons about labeling ourselves with preexisting conditions.

You see, we often underestimate the power of our bodies to communicate with us. We can be quick to explain away new symptoms, attributing them to existing health issues. It's easy to dismiss warning signs, thinking they're just part of the same old struggle. However, this phase of my life taught me a crucial lesson - never to overlook or downplay the signals your body sends. It's a lesson that would reshape the trajectory of my journey, reminding me that even the darkest clouds can have a silver lining.

More often than not, having a preexisting condition might lead you down a confusing rabbit hole when you encounter new health concerns. It's a lesson that I, myself, learned the hard way. Let me emphasize just how crucial it is to approach medications, treatments, and surgeries with caution in today's world of booming healthcare, where profit often takes precedence over genuine well-being. My journey has taught me that it's essential to be an informed advocate for your health. Our healthcare system has evolved into a thriving industry, with many individuals undergoing unnecessary procedures, all under the guise of pursuing good health. The truth is that the very nature of my experience underlines the irony of this situation. Neither of my potentially terminal diseases would have ever come to light through routine screening because I was simply considered too young for such conditions.

Take a moment to let that sink in - if I had disregarded the worsening symptoms of breast cancer, I would have been confronted by this insidious disease long before I reached the age when routine mammograms are typically recommended. It's a stark reminder that life doesn't always neatly adhere to the schedules and guidelines we've come to rely on.

In retrospect, my journey through the healthcare system revealed that we often need to be our own advocates. It's a story that underscores the importance of listening to our bodies and not easily dismissing symptoms. Had I not been persistent in seeking answers, my story could have had a tragically different ending. It's a testament to the need for individuals to be proactive about their health, to question assumptions, and to demand thorough evaluations when something just doesn't feel right.

This phase of my life was a turning point, not only in my health but in my perspective on healthcare itself. The experiences I encountered during this period became a driving force behind my mission to share my story, urging others to take their health into their own hands. Life, as I've come to understand, is a delicate dance between chance and choice. And it's in those moments of choice, like the one where I chose to confront my symptoms head-on, that our destinies can be shaped in ways we never expected.

Thankfully, I heeded the silent whispers of my intuition and persevered. Consider it a cautionary tale, a reminder to trust your gut and listen to your body when something new and worrisome arises. My life had been marked by a distinct lack of a mother figure or anyone reliable to turn to for support, which often left me feeling adrift in the turbulent sea of existence.

Growing up with a close family member struggling with mental health issues, it became almost routine to question my own sanity. The pervasive self-doubt that lingers in such an environment can erode your confidence and cast shadows on even the most mundane aspects of life. I found myself second-guessing everything, except for one undeniable fact – the protrusion in my left breast, which stubbornly continued to grow. I can't help but admit that during this period, I often questioned my own sanity. It's a feeling that can consume you and make you wonder if you're losing your grip on reality. But amidst this internal turmoil, one undeniable truth remained: the large lump that had taken up residence in my left breast. It was a tangible, physical reminder that I wasn't merely imagining things.

After enduring three visits to my primary doctor, my concerns about this growing, mysterious lump could no longer be dismissed. What initially might have seemed like an ordinary cyst had morphed into a source of mounting apprehension. It was time for action, a reality check of sorts.

Amidst the cacophony of self-doubt and uncertainty, the decision was made to conduct a biopsy. It felt like the most rational step to take, a way to finally ascertain the true nature of this "common" cyst that had silently, yet relentlessly, invaded my body. This was the turning point where I transitioned from passive concern to proactive self-advocacy. It's a reminder that sometimes, you have to be your own advocate, even when doubts cast their shadows. And it's also a testament to the incredible strength that can be summoned when faced with the unknown. The journey continued, but now, I was determined to chart my own course.

The day for my biopsy had finally arrived, and I couldn't help but feel a mix of excitement and nervousness. My insurance had approved the procedure, and it was carefully scheduled. As I walked into the medical facility, I pondered what this test might uncover about the mysterious lump in my left breast. Would it be just another medical procedure, or would it reveal something deeper and more profound?

Once inside, the clinical environment surrounded me, and I realized I was at a pivotal moment in my journey. I had to summon my courage and trust in the medical professionals who were about to guide me through this crucial process. The procedure held the promise of unraveling the mysteries that had been haunting me, and I was ready to face whatever came next. I exchanged my clothing for the open-facing half gown, which always manages to make you feel a tad vulnerable. As I lay down on the cold, sterile bed, I reflected on the road that had brought me to this point. I was here to find out the truth, and I was determined to confront it head-on.

The medical team meticulously prepared the area on the side of my left breast for the ultrasound-guided biopsy. Their experienced hands moved with precision as they cleaned and sterilized the area. It was a poignant reminder of the balance between science and humanity, where skilled professionals worked tirelessly to bring clarity to the unknown.

The biopsy procedure went relatively smoothly, just as I expected, although there was indeed some mild discomfort. Little did I know at that moment that the phrase "mild discomfort" would become a recurring theme in my journey, almost turning into a sort of dark humor as I encountered more challenging aspects of my treatment. It was a peek behind the curtain of medical terminology that often understates the true experience of patients.

As I lay there, the radiologist, during the biopsy, kept up a casual conversation. It was a strange contrast to the tense anticipation I was feeling. She shared her belief that this was likely just a common, benign cyst, the kind that many women experience, and she advised me not to worry too much until the procedure was completed. The words flowed from her like a reassuring river, soothing the anxious thoughts that had been racing through my mind. It was almost as if her casual banter was designed to keep my mind off the procedure itself. I appreciated her attempt to put me at ease, even if it was just for a short while.

Once the biopsy was done, the radiologist's confidence seemed to soar. She assured me that everything had gone as expected, reinforcing her belief that it was indeed a cyst. Her words were like a lifeline in that moment, a beacon of hope amid the sea of uncertainty. As she concluded, she kindly reminded me that my personal physician would soon have the results in hand.

I took a few moments to gather myself, having dressed again after the biopsy procedure. I returned to the waiting room, not out of necessity, but more to find a quiet space where I could be alone with my thoughts. It wasn't so much the actual procedure that I needed to decompress from but rather the staggering reality that had just washed over me. Sitting there, I was enveloped by the stillness of the waiting room, a stark contrast to the whirlwind of emotions churning within me. I was given the freedom to leave, yet something compelled me to stay and contemplate the weight of the situation. It was an opportunity to let the enormity of the moment truly sink in.

It wasn't just a medical procedure I had undergone; it was the stark realization that I might be facing breast cancer. The knowledge that my life, as I currently knew it, was on the precipice of a profound and irrevocable change weighed heavily on my mind. The future had suddenly become uncertain, and it was a lot to absorb. During those precious minutes, I sat there in introspection, reflecting on the twists and turns life could take. Emotions of fear and anxiety intermingled with hope, creating a complex tapestry of thoughts. It was a moment of reckoning, a pause in the narrative of my life to come to terms with the unknown.

In this unexpected interlude in the waiting room, I realized that my journey was at a crossroads. The road ahead was uncertain, and the path would be different from anything I had traversed before. The words of the radiologist, her assurance, became a glimmer of hope that I held onto as I faced the upcoming challenges.

Walking through life with the specter of a potentially terminal disease is a peculiar and unsettling experience. It's a path laden with uncertainty, one that demands a level of resilience that I never knew I possessed. The weight of it all, the knowledge that my health was in jeopardy, hung over me like a persistent storm cloud. Yet, I had to find the strength to hold it together, not only for my own sake but for the well-being of my family and my own sanity.

Staring down the barrel of a year-long treatment plan was no small feat. The gravity of my situation became all too real as I contemplated the long road ahead. A 26-week chemotherapy regimen lay before me, a challenging journey that would test not only my physical endurance but my mental fortitude as well. My doctor's concerns added to the already heavy burden I carried. It was evident that they worried about whether I could endure the rigors of this extended treatment. The uncertainty of the outcome hung over every discussion and appointment. It was a stark reminder that my journey was fraught with both hope and trepidation, a balancing act between optimism and the harsh reality of my medical condition.

There was no room for me to dwell on my situation; life moved at a relentless pace. My oncologist, a no-nonsense head of the department, had a reputation for being strict and old-school in her approach to treatment. She held a belief that didn't align with the modern use of ports for chemotherapy administration. To her, these ports represented a constant source of infection, and she harbored deep concerns about the risk of me being hospitalized due to a port-related infection during my treatment.

This was a stark reminder of the harsh realities of my medical journey. My oncologist's approach was rooted in a desire to safeguard my health and minimize potential complications. It was a reflection of the medical ethos she adhered to, one that prioritized patient well-being above all else. As I navigated through the challenging landscape of my treatment, I couldn't help but acknowledge the wisdom in her old-school approach. It was an example of how the medical field had evolved and how different doctors had contrasting perspectives on what was best for their patients.

My oncologist's decision was clear - I would commence my treatment without a port, and any further consideration would be made if necessary. This old-school approach meant that I'd be navigating the world of chemotherapy with the use of large cannulas, which are more substantial than what most patients typically encounter with traditional intravenous therapy. These cannulas are essentially the tubes inserted into the veins to facilitate the administration of intravenous therapy.

The process of undergoing chemotherapy was far from ordinary. To minimize discomfort, the routine involved receiving a lidocaine injection in the area where the chemotherapy would be administered. In my case, it was my forearms, with weekly alternations between the two arms. The lidocaine injection did cause some mild pain, but fortunately, I found the strength to endure it.

Ironically, as I went through my treatments, I discovered that the lidocaine injections turned out to be the most challenging part. After my second or third session, I decided to skip a minor inconvenience in the grand scheme of things. For me, the lidocaine injections brought a temporary burning sensation that, oddly enough, proved to be more discomforting than the actual insertion of the cannula. So, after a few sessions, I made a conscious decision to skip these injections for the remainder of my treatment. This choice not only lessened the physical discomfort but also helped me mentally prepare for each session. Knowing that I'd only experience one "poke" during each treatment brought a sense of predictability to an otherwise unpredictable process.

My unconventional approach became my personal coping mechanism. It allowed me to navigate the world of chemotherapy with a measure of control and predictability. While it may not have been the conventional path, it was a choice I made to find comfort in an otherwise challenging journey. Top of Form

One of the silver linings of this decision was that I managed to avoid the need for the insertion of a port. In the grand scheme of things, this was a small victory, but it was a testament to the choices and adaptations I was willing to make as I fought my way through the tough terrain of chemotherapy. It was a reminder that sometimes, the path to recovery isn't a straight line, and the decisions we make along the way can have a significant impact on our journey.

My first chemotherapy treatment unfolded much as expected, but it took a distressing turn when I found myself in need of emergency treatment for heart failure, a side effect related to Adriamycin, also known as doxorubicin. It was a harrowing experience, and the subsequent brief hospitalization left me shaken and vulnerable.

Returning for my second treatment, I faced a lower dose of Adriamycin, administered with great caution to prevent a recurrence of the cardiac incident. With each completed treatment, there was a palpable sense of relief. It was as though I had reached a milestone, one step closer to the finish line in this marathon of a treatment plan.

The need for hospitalization within 24 hours of my first chemotherapy session was a devastating blow. As I lay in hospital bed, staring at the ceiling in the dimly lit room, I grappled with the overwhelming emotions that swirled around me. In that moment, it became apparent that I had no choice but to find a way to disconnect my emotions from the daunting treatment plan if I were to endure. It was as if a revelation struck me during that solitary moment in the hospital room. I understood that in order to survive this ordeal, I needed to sever the ties that bound my mind to negative outcomes. I resolved to shift my focus away from worrying about the future and fixate instead on the daily tasks that lay before me. My strategy was to take one day at a time and avoid gazing too far ahead on the calendar.

The proposed calendar for my treatment journey was a daunting one. It stretched over 26 weeks of chemotherapy, with brief breaks to prepare for multiple surgeries and another set of breaks to allow for post-surgery healing. Following that, there were an additional 9 weeks of daily radiation therapy looming on the horizon. The enormity of this timeline felt almost insurmountable, and it left me wrestling with the weight of uncertainty.

In that pivotal moment, I made a profound decision. I chose to relinquish the burden of worry and surrender it all to a higher power. It was as though I lifted the heavy load from my shoulders and handed it back to God, trusting in a force greater than myself to guide the way. This act of surrender wasn't an admission of defeat but rather a conscious choice to let go of the fear and anxiety that had been clouding my path.

As I gave it all back, there was a sense of release, an unburdening of my mind. It was as though I had cleared the clutter and noise that had been consuming my thoughts. With this newfound clarity, I could redirect my focus, channeling my energy into the physical aspects of my healing journey from breast cancer.

Faith undeniably plays a significant role in the journey of cancer care. I firmly believe in its impact, and my experience reaffirmed this belief. Leaning on a higher power during my treatment brought a sense of solace and reduced my worries. It's a somewhat indescribable feeling, akin to entrusting the bulk of your workload to someone willing to help.

In the beginning, I was somewhat naive, believing that I could manage everything on my own. Being fiercely independent had served me well in many aspects of life, but cancer and its demanding treatment would put my self-reliance to the test. I quickly found myself reevaluating what independence meant to me.

It became apparent that accepting help was not a sign of weakness but a necessary part of my healing journey. This was a turning point where I began to allow others to share the burden of my worries. Whether it was assistance with meals or rides to medical appointments, there were individuals who generously stepped up to support both me and my family during this challenging period.

The journey through treatment proved to be the most challenging endeavor of my life. It wasn't just the physical toll of enduring the unpleasant side effects but the emotional weight that came with it. The pain, the moments of hopelessness, and the lurking fear of whether I would ultimately survive cancer all combined to create an overwhelming storm. The completion of my first round of chemotherapy marked a significant milestone. Those initial four months of treatment were behind me, and somehow, against all odds, I had persevered. Chemo had proven effective; the tumor was shrinking, my heart and veins held up, and my mental health remained stable. Yet, in the realm of cancer, there remained a multitude of unknowns. Instead of allowing these uncertainties to consume me, I chose to channel my worries into prayer.

Before each treatment, procedure, scan, or surgery, I would offer up my prayers. I also reached out to others, asking for their prayers and support. It was as if the collective force of these prayers would carry me through the toughest of times. I prayed for strength, for courage, and for the tenacity to fight through this formidable adversary. In a lighthearted way, I would even pray to "stay too mean to die," a sentiment that was born out of the sheer disbelief of receiving such an unfathomable diagnosis. After all, young women weren't supposed to get breast cancer.

After a brief respite, my chemotherapy journey continued with a 12-week course of once-a-week infusions of Taxol. However, this phase of treatment also had its share of harrowing moments. I found myself hospitalized once more, facing life-threatening adverse reactions to the treatment. Fortunately, after spending eight days in the hospital, I regained enough strength to return home and resume the treatment without further incident.

Throughout this challenging phase, the power of prayers from my community continued to be a source of solace and strength. It was evident that the combination of medical treatment and collective prayers was working, and I felt a deep sense of gratitude toward everyone who rallied around me. My friends and community offered more than just their prayers; they provided meals, rides to treatment, and unwavering support. It was a tremendous comfort to experience such care, especially since my earlier years had been marked by self-reliance. As a child, I had borne the weight of my own care and often that of my younger half-siblings as well.

Accepting help as an adult was initially a challenge, but the side effects of my treatment left me with no choice. Taxol, in particular, was a long and arduous journey. The excruciating pain it inflicted felt as if every nerve ending in my body was ablaze. Even the most potent pain relievers offered only partial relief. It was during this phase that I began to doubt my ability to make it through the treatment. For the first time, despite the two previous serious hospitalizations, I felt that I might not survive this battle. I confided in my husband about my fears, expressing my belief that I might not make it. His response was to offer reassurance, patting my bald head and encouraging me to take another pain pill and rest. Looking back, I understand that it was his way of coping, of trying to maintain some semblance of normalcy in a world turned upside down by the upheaval of cancer.

In the midst of the turmoil, I recognized that a strong and healthy relationship could be an anchor during these turbulent times. If anything, cancer had revealed the resilience of our bond. It was during the darkest moments of this journey that the strength of our connection truly shone.

Following the successful completion of the proposed chemotherapy regimens, I finally had a brief respite from treatment, a month to catch my breath, and prepare for the next chapter of my journey: surgery. Little did I know that surgery would evolve into a series of surgeries. My staging had been reevaluated, and I was now categorized as Stage 3, eliminating the possibility of a double mastectomy. Additionally, I had tested negative for the BRCA gene, which meant there was no medical rationale for a radical mastectomy. This shift in my treatment plan was accompanied by the comforting news that my prognosis had improved considerably, thanks to the successful shrinkage of the tumor through chemotherapy.

During this break, I began to notice the signs of my former self returning. My hair started to grow back, symbolizing a rekindling of life and vitality. It was as though my body and mind were gradually regaining their strength, and I found inspiration in these subtle transformations. Alongside medical treatment, I leaned into prayer and meditation, embracing them as powerful tools for healing my body from cancer. This holistic approach not only nurtured my physical well-being but also fortified my mental resilience.

The month passed swiftly, and before I knew it, I was sitting in the office of my new surgeon. We went over the extensive checklist of preparations needed for my upcoming left-sided lumpectomy. This surgical procedure was the next step in my journey, and I approached it with a mix of hope and determination. Little did I know that it would be a pivotal moment in my battle against breast cancer, marking another chapter in my story of resilience and recovery.

The day of my surgery arrived, and I was a bundle of nerves. What no one really tells you about this whole process is how the steroids can affect you. They make you feel all sorts of emotions, intensifying the already present pain and uncertainty. It's not the greatest combination, to say the least.

My emotions felt raw, and I was in excruciating pain from the procedure of being blue dye mapped for the lumpectomy, an essential step to ensure they could achieve clear margins around the cancerous area. Picture me, nearly bald, donned in a hospital gown, an IV in place, and bandages on the left side of my chest from the dye mapping. To top it off, my surgery had been delayed. That's when my anesthesiologist strolled into the room.

Now, I must emphasize that my entire medical team was truly amazing, and every one of them played a vital role in saving my life. However, on this particular day, my anesthesiologist became the unwitting recipient of my frustration. I couldn't help but question his competence, half-jokingly, asking if it was his first day on the job as he let me keep my sunglasses on while I lay on the surgical table during pre-surgery preparations. Try to imagine the scene: there I was, lying on a cold steel table, topless, with dark sunglasses on, waiting for surgery to remove the cancerous tumor from my body. As my surgeon walked in and noticed the peculiar sight, she inquired, "Why is she still wearing her sunglasses?" directed at the anesthesiologist. Looking back on that moment, I can't help but find some humor in it. Despite the frustration I felt at the time, it provided a much-needed moment of comic relief for all of us.

The surgery proceeded without any further incident, which was a tremendous relief. Meanwhile, my husband had been patiently waiting in the hospital's waiting area throughout the procedure, anxious for updates. He had no idea about the events unfolding beyond those surgical doors. At one point, a tall, visibly frustrated doctor emerged from the operating room, and my husband couldn't help but wonder if this doctor had been a part of my surgical team.

After a few more hours of anticipation, I was finally given the green light to go home. My surgeon declared the surgery a success, describing it as excellent. When I was reunited with my husband, I had to explain the source of my earlier frustration with the anesthesiologist. He chuckled and shared that he, too, had encountered the same frustrated doctor afterward. I couldn't help but feel a tad guilty, but at that point, I was simply too exhausted to dwell on it any longer.

My focus now had to shift entirely to healing from surgery. However, just two days later, our world was shaken by devastating news. The lab report on the tumor removal indicated that clear margins had not been achieved during the lumpectomy on my chest. In simpler terms, it meant that traces of cancer still lingered. My surgeon acted swiftly, scheduling a repeat surgery for the following week. The news was devastating, and fear began to tighten its grip. I found myself consumed by worries about whether the cancer had spread elsewhere in my body. Soon, a fever developed, forcing the surgery to be postponed for two more weeks.

After receiving the disheartening news about the failed surgery and dealing with a week of tears, accompanied by a persistent fever and the painful healing process from the initial procedure, I knew I had to find a way to quell the creeping fear and doubt. I turned to prayer, seeking solace in my faith, and I asked for more prayers from those around me. It was a time to refocus my energy on the love and support of my family and friends. The two weeks passed slowly, but they brought about a significant change. My fever had subsided, and my blood counts showed improvement. Emotionally, I was in a better place. Thanks to the power of prayer and meditation, my spirits had been lifted from the depths of despair that had followed the initial surgery. Hope began to take root, and I started to believe that the next surgery would be the one to finally rid my body of cancer.

The day of the surgery arrived, and I went into it with renewed optimism. This time, everything went smoothly, and there was no hint of negativity surrounding the procedure. The wait for the results felt like an eternity, but when the news finally came, it was exactly what I had been hoping for – my margins were clear, and the cancer was gone. I was granted another four weeks of respite from treatment to heal from the two lumpectomies. My spirit felt renewed, and I started to embrace a newfound sense of hope. My family relished this break, and life began to feel normal once more. It was a time of restoration, recovery, and the resurgence of hope, and I cherished every moment of it.

As time swiftly passed, it was time to embark on the last phase of my cancer treatment journey, which entailed reporting to my new radiologist. Throughout this entire process, I cannot express enough gratitude to all our friends, family, acquaintances, and even strangers who prayed for us and offered their help. I genuinely believe that when someone prays for you, those prayers are heard by a higher power, and the energy is transformed into your well-being.

Just when I had started to feel a semblance of normalcy returning, the last part of my treatment, a grueling nine-week daily radiation schedule, loomed before me. I couldn't help but resent the process of getting radiation markers tattooed on my body. My radiologist tried to lighten the mood, suggesting that I think of them as freckles. However, my dismay remained because nobody has blue freckles, right?

Daily, I reported for radiation therapy, and the burns gradually intensified over time. My skin around the treatment area began to take on a dark, almost blackened appearance. My entire chest felt scorched, but there was a silver lining – my hair had started to grow in more fully. What's more, it was incredibly curly, quite the change from my naturally super straight hair. I was both amazed and amused by this unexpected transformation, a tangible reminder of the resilience I had displayed throughout my cancer journey.

There I was, sitting with my short curly hair and radiation burns on my chest, trying my best to look and feel normal. I had almost become unrecognizable to myself. This final leg of my treatment journey was proving to be just as challenging as the rest. What people often don't talk about is the emotional toll of treatment itself. When you couple that with the constant worry of cancer and the financial hardships that can follow while still trying to be present in your own life, it can be beyond draining. That's why prayer and meditation remained consistent pillars for me to lean on during my treatment and in every aspect of my life.

What I hope you take away from my journey is that many unexpected negative things can happen, and yet you can still find a positive outcome. I thought I would die several times over during my year-long treatment plan, facing numerous life-threatening complications. But somehow, I persevered and made it through all of it, returning to excellent health. I recently celebrated my 12-year anniversary of being breast cancer-free, and it's a testament to the strength of the human spirit and the support of faith. As I reflect on it all, there's one thing that remains constant – my ability to laugh. I once joked that I must be "too mean to die" and that humor has been a source of resilience and strength throughout the years. It's a reminder that even in the face of adversity, there can be moments of joy and laughter, and they are worth celebrating.

Radiation therapy continued for a few more weeks, but with each passing day, I could feel the finish line drawing closer. Finally, on December 31, 2011, I officially completed that monumental, overwhelming year-long treatment plan. I was not only free of treatment but also free of cancer. It was a feeling of being unbreakable, a sense of happiness that filled my entire being. It was a powerful reminder of the impact of both prayer and modern medicine.

The moral of my story, one that I hope resonates with anyone facing a similar journey, is the importance of leaning into prayer and seeking help from friends and family. It's about giving your burdens and worries back to a higher power. This combination of inner solitude and the comforting presence of loved ones can work wonders. It can free your body from the weight of worry and allow you to triumph over cancer.

CHAPTER 6
ALOHA AND RUNNING BLIND

After completing my year-long battle with Stage III Triple Negative Breast cancer, I thought I had successfully turned a new page in my life. I was in the process of settling into the revamped version of myself, a person who had conquered an insidious disease. However, my journey to recovery was far from over, and I was still grappling with a host of lingering side effects. The uncertainty of how long some of these effects would persist and whether they would eventually become a permanent part of my life loomed like a shadow over my newfound sense of wellness.

My oncologist continued to play a vital role in my life, conducting regular check-ups and biannual scans to ensure that the cancer had not stealthily resurfaced anywhere in my body. Life was seemingly back on track, and I cherished every moment of my newfound health and happiness. But, as life often reminds us, things can change in the blink of an eye.

The first signs of trouble manifested in the form of relentless headaches, sneaking into my daily life at an alarming speed. These unwelcome guests were like storm clouds on a sunny day, darkening my world with throbbing pain. To make matters worse, my eyes had become incredibly sensitive to even the gentlest rays of light. It was as if I was living in a perpetual eclipse, needing to shield my eyes from the world. My sunglasses became an integral part of my daily attire, a constant companion that helped me face the day.

Yet, I tried to navigate through life as inconspicuously as possible, pretending as though my choice of eyewear was a mere fashion statement rather than a necessity. I didn't want anyone to know the truth: that I was concealing a hidden burden, a brain tumor that had emerged to challenge my newfound sense of victory.

Only a select few of my closest friends were privy to the original diagnosis, and they knew the secret behind my ever-present sunglasses. I shared this information with them, not as a plea for sympathy but as a means of explaining why I had become inseparable from my shades. I wanted them to understand the pain and fear I was facing daily.

The fear of misinterpretation weighed heavily on my mind. I was terrified that people who didn't know my situation might mistake my sunglasses for a disguise for inebriation or some illicit substance. The thought of being judged or misunderstood added an extra layer of complexity to an already challenging journey.

Addiction was a concept that had never cast its shadow over my life until it unexpectedly entered my world amidst the most challenging phase of my radiation treatment. It was a period in which I was grappling with excruciating pain and a heavy burden of illness. During those dark days, a friend voiced a concern that caught me completely off guard. She believed, or rather feared, that I was on the precipice of developing an addiction to the pain medication I was prescribed.

Little did she know, my situation was far from ordinary. My chest bore the evidence of a brutal struggle, etched with blackened third-degree burns – a painful testament to the toll cancer had taken on my body. These agonizing burns were just one layer of the physical torment I endured, layered atop the excruciating bone pain that had already been a constant companion, a relentless reminder of my previous Taxol treatment. The pain I endured was like a relentless tempest that had no regard for the fragility of my being.

Cancer is an affliction that not only tests the physical limits of the body but also relentlessly erodes one's emotional and mental fortitude. It's a battle for which no one can fully prepare, a relentless storm that uproots the life you once knew. It's a challenge that you confront daily, not knowing what lies ahead yet summoning the courage to face it head-on.

When my friend finally saw the harrowing sight of those third-degree burns on my chest, her gasp of horror echoed through the room. It was then that she truly comprehended the depth of my pain and suffering. The interaction served as a turning point in our relationship, as she realized the immense gravity of what I was enduring. It was a stark reminder that life could be profoundly complex, throwing unexpected challenges at us, but it also revealed the transformative power of empathy and understanding.

During my tumultuous journey through cancer treatment, some friendships underwent a metamorphosis. They either transformed into a source of unwavering support, growing stronger in the face of adversity, or, in some cases, faded into the background. The ebb and flow of friendships during such a trying period was a testament to life's capricious nature. Just when you believe you have your path figured out, life can alter it dramatically, leading you to places you could never have anticipated.

As I reflect on the twists and turns of my cancer journey, I am filled with gratitude for every experience, both the painful and the heartwarming. Each trial and tribulation ultimately molded me into a stronger, more resilient individual, preparing me for the next unforeseen battle that awaited me – the daunting challenge of an inoperable brain tumor.

The day the results of my brain MRI came in was one etched in my memory, not for any joyous reasons but for the shattering news it brought. My previously diagnosed brain tumor, which I had hoped was under control, unveiled its relentless nature. The report was grim; the tumor had not only persisted but was now growing at an alarming pace. It was as if it had unleashed a hidden fury within me.

This devastating revelation prompted my primary doctor to make the difficult decision to refer me for further evaluation. It was time to confront the reality of the situation head-on, a reality that was anything but comforting. The medical experts confirmed the dire prognosis, confirming my worst fears.

The tumor had taken up residence in the center of my left ventricle, a strategic location that allowed it to exert pressure on every area it touched. The gravity of the situation was palpable, and the cruel irony was that traditional surgery, the usual go-to solution in such cases, was ruled out as an option. To go under the knife would mean slicing through too much healthy brain tissue, a move that would likely be as lethal as the tumor itself. The treatment options I had hoped for seemed to crumble before my eyes.

At that moment, I was faced with an agonizing truth – there were no immediate treatment options available. The room felt heavy with the weight of despair as the medical professionals delivered this somber verdict. The future appeared bleak, like an unending night that refused to yield to the dawn.

The doctors' words echoed in my mind, urging me to consider an unthinkable task: getting my affairs in order. It was a grim suggestion, a reminder that the relentless march of time could be tragically unpredictable. The tumor's growth was a time bomb, ticking away the moments of my life, and if it took an unexpected turn, it could snatch life from me without warning.

As I grappled with this harsh reality, I found myself in a place of contemplation. The uncertainty of life had never been more vivid, and the fragility of our existence had never felt more real. It was a time to reflect, to cherish the moments that remained, and to prepare for the inevitable unknown that lay ahead.

After that fateful appointment, I somehow managed to make it back home, a journey that felt like a blur against the backdrop of San Diego's relentless rush-hour traffic. It was a city that had become my home nearly a decade ago, a place where my husband had accepted a job with the Scripps Health organization. Little did I know back then that this very organization would later play a pivotal role in my life, not just as a source of employment for my husband but as the lifeline that would eventually save me when breast cancer reared its ugly head.

As I navigated the familiar streets, I couldn't help but reflect on the irony of it all. The same organization that had welcomed us to this vibrant city would soon become the epicenter of my battle against a formidable adversary. I had been diagnosed with breast cancer, a diagnosis that had led me down a treacherous path of treatments and tests, and now, it seemed, it had brought me to the most dreaded crossroads.

What lay ahead was a stark and disheartening realization. The treatments, the countless doctor appointments, the unwavering support of my brilliant husband, all of it had brought me to this moment. I couldn't help but feel an eerie sense of calm as I contemplated the somber truth: there were no more treatment options available to save my life. It was as if I had reached the end of a perilous road, and there was no turning back.

The gravity of the situation weighed on me as I considered that my doctors, no matter how skilled and dedicated, could not offer a miraculous solution this time. Even my brilliant husband, who had been my unwavering pillar of support throughout this journey, couldn't fix what lay ahead. It was a reality that I had to face, no matter how painful or daunting it seemed.

In the midst of this overwhelming uncertainty, I found solace in the deep bond that had formed between us and the city of San Diego. It was a city that had witnessed the highs and lows of our lives, a place where we had built our home and our dreams. It was a place where I had encountered the darkest challenge of my life, and yet, it was also a place where I had found unexpected sources of strength and support.

As I gazed into the mirror, the reflection staring back at me held the weight of an impending fate. I felt like a dead woman walking, an eerie sensation that lingered in the corners of my mind. Despite the undeniable strength that seemed to radiate from my appearance, I couldn't ignore the incessant blinking of my eyes, a subconscious countdown to what I could only perceive as my untimely demise.

In the harsh, unrelenting glare of the bedroom lights, my blinking eyes mirrored the uncertainty that had become a relentless companion. It was as if my own body was playing a cruel trick on me, signaling that I could drop dead at any given moment. The threat of sudden, unpredictable seizures hung over me like a menacing storm cloud, a stark reminder of the fragility of life that I had come to accept.

With the impending risk of seizures looming over me, I made a painful yet necessary decision – I could no longer drive. The keys to my car, once a symbol of freedom and independence, now sat idly on the kitchen counter. It was a sobering realization that I had to relinquish control over yet another aspect of my life.

The gravity of my situation continued to unravel as I faced another dire warning. The prospect of going completely blind was a haunting reality that I had to confront. I had already been diagnosed as functionally blind, a result of the relentless brain swelling that was affecting my optic nerve. It was as if the world was slowly slipping through my fingers, one ray of light at a time.

In the midst of these overwhelming challenges, I made a choice to release my worries, a burden that had grown heavier with each passing day. I turned to faith, to a higher power, and decided to surrender my fears and anxieties to the divine. It was a recurring act, one that I had performed countless times throughout my journey, a testament to the enduring power of faith and resilience.

With the specter of my own mortality looming over me, I couldn't help but acknowledge the harsh reality – the odds were stacked against me. It was a strangely liberating feeling, one that came from the acceptance that the battle had reached its end. The fight had concluded, and I was left to contemplate the life I had led.

The feeling of having lived in survival mode for such an extended period was like a relentless storm that had swept through my life. Yet, amidst the challenges and hardships, I learned to face life with a dash of humor. I would often chuckle to myself, recognizing that despite the tumultuous journey, I hadn't grown up to be a kleptomaniac or a paranoid schizophrenic. It was a testament to the resilience of the human spirit and the ability to find humor in even the darkest of times.

My life had been a series of twists and turns, triumphs and tribulations. I couldn't help but acknowledge that while I had faced many hurdles, I had also been fortunate enough to taste success in various facets of life. I had excelled in many areas, except perhaps in the realm of marriage. It was a truth that I carried with a certain degree of regret, having been married three times in my life, two of those unions occurring before I had even reached the age of twenty. The circumstances that had led me to these choices were complex, including the turmoil of my mother's mental illness, which had cast a shadow over our lives and left us homeless at times.

In retrospect, my journey appeared to be a relentless series of hard-fought challenges, each one met with determination and the unshakable belief that education would be my passport to success. I set my sights on becoming a lawyer, a dream that drove me to attend a Certified Paralegal program, allowing me to support myself as I aspired to achieve my goals. I knew that I had to be resourceful and that the path to success would require unwavering commitment and a readiness to adapt to changing circumstances.

Upon graduation, however, life had different plans for me. I found myself compelled to pivot and shift my focus. Nursing, it seemed, was the next chapter in my life. It was a decision that wasn't made lightly, but it was a choice that I embraced with open arms. Nursing school was a challenging endeavor, and yet I emerged from it with a sense of accomplishment, a diploma in hand, and the knowledge that I was prepared to make a difference in the world of healthcare.

A decade of a fulfilling nursing career followed a path that brought me closer to the purpose I had been seeking. I reveled in the opportunity to help others to be a guiding light in their moments of need. It was in the world of nursing that I discovered the path that would lead me forward.

In a life filled with uncertainty and hardships, I also had my share of serendipitous moments. It was in these moments that destiny seemed to guide my way. I had the good fortune of meeting my current partner, and our connection was nothing short of fate. We've spent twenty-five remarkable years together, and he is more than just a partner; he is my soulmate. It was as though the universe had conspired to bring us together, and in his presence, I found the strength and the support to navigate the challenges that lay ahead. He became not only a partner but also a lifeline, a constant reminder that even in the darkest times, there can be a glimmer of hope and a chance at a brighter future.

In the wake of completing my grueling cancer treatment, my spirit was alive with a newfound sense of hope and determination. The world seemed to open its arms, and the possibilities were endless. At that time, life had yet to deliver the crushing blow of my brain tumor diagnosis, and my husband and I were planning a grand adventure. It was an escapade that we had envisioned for the better part of ten months, a celebration of life's resilience and the desire to make the most of the time we had left.

The plan was ambitious, a grand journey that would span thirty days. We would set sail from the bustling city of Los Angeles, bound for the Samoan Islands, and from there, we'd embark on a voyage that would take us all around the enchanting Hawaiian Islands. Our adventure would culminate with a mesmerizing cruise through the idyllic waters of French Polynesia before making our way back to the shores of California.

It was a dream come true, a reminder that life, even in its most challenging moments, could offer remarkable opportunities. We were set to explore pristine beaches, navigate crystal-clear waters, and immerse ourselves in the diverse cultures of these beautiful island paradises. The anticipation of this epic journey filled our hearts with joy, and it became a symbol of the strength and resilience that had carried us through the darkest days of my illness.

This grand adventure, however, would prove to be more than just a vacation. It would become a pivotal moment, a turning point in our lives. It was during this voyage that my husband and I made a decision that would forever alter the course of our future. We decided to move to Hawaii to embrace its beauty and serenity for the remainder of my life.

Six months after we had set sail on that memorable cruise, I found myself stepping onto the shores of Hawaii, my new home. It was a decision made with both hope and a tinge of melancholy. The breast cancer that had once threatened to consume me had been vanquished, but the shadow of my original prognosis still loomed, foretelling that I wouldn't survive another five years. Moreover, the ominous presence of the brain tumor added an even greater sense of urgency, with doctors predicting that it might claim my life within the year.

In Hawaii, I found solace in the embrace of the lush landscapes, the soothing ocean waves, and the vibrant culture that surrounded me. It became a place where I could truly appreciate the precious moments of life, plan for my eventual departure, and create lasting memories with my loved ones.

The move to Hawaii unfolded with unexpected swiftness, a whirlwind of decisions and farewells that saw us parting with most of our possessions. My husband, ever the devoted companion, took the plunge into retirement by giving notice on his job. We dove headfirst into the pursuit of a temporary place to call home in the Hawaiian paradise, fully aware that my stay there might be brief, given the foreboding prognosis associated with my brain tumor.

The transition to island life was smoother than we could have ever anticipated, almost as if the universe was conspiring to bring us peace and tranquility. Everything seemed to fall seamlessly into place, and it was almost too easy to embrace the serenity of Hawaii, a far cry from the tumultuous journey we had embarked upon.

Despite my newfound island bliss, the sense of responsibility tugged at me. I felt compelled to find one last doctor to monitor my brain tumor, partly to appease the concerns of my family and friends. The move to Hawaii, though filled with hope, could not, I knew, magically cure all my problems. I embarked on this journey with a sense of surrender, deciding to cast my worries to the wind, trusting in a higher power.

My conversations with God, which had evolved over time, now resembled conversations with an old friend. The words spoken in those quiet moments were raw and unfiltered, expressions of the deep well of emotions that had welled up within me. It was in this state of surrender and vulnerability that something magical transpired.

I was led to the office of a brilliant Vietnamese neurosurgeon, a man of unwavering confidence. He entered the room, poised and determined, radiating an air of competence that both reassured and unnerved me. His words cut through the uncertainty that had enveloped my life. He outlined a proposed treatment plan, one that carried with it the power to either obliterate the tumor or potentially rob me of my ability to walk or talk. It was a stark choice, one that felt like a test of my courage and my resolve.

In the face of this proposition, fury welled up within me. I found myself telling the doctor in no uncertain terms that I did not wish to hear the adverse reactions ever again. It was as if the weight of my experiences had given rise to a newfound defiance. I had spent years preparing for the worst, ready to face any challenge that life could throw at me. Yet, in that moment, life had thrown me an unexpected curveball, and I was left to confront a choice that was beyond any I had imagined.

Leaving that neurosurgeon's office, my mind was a tumultuous sea of doubt and uncertainty. Had I fallen prey to island fever, conjuring up the entire appointment within my imagination? I couldn't help but question the reliability of my own senses. Frustration welled up within me, and I found myself raising my voice to the heavens, urging God to cease playing games with my fate. It was a moment of raw vulnerability and desperation, and I knew that I needed to share the events of that appointment with my husband.

As I recounted the meeting with the neurosurgeon, a glimmer of clarity began to emerge. It was as if the pieces of a cosmic puzzle were falling into place. Had God, in His mysterious ways, revealed to me a path to save my own life? Perhaps the purpose of bringing me to Hawaii was not to be a final chapter but a new beginning. The island had beckoned me, not as a place to meet my end, but as a sanctuary of hope, where life could be rekindled.

With this newfound understanding, a profound sense of gratitude washed over me. I was meant to live, and the path ahead was one I would embrace with open arms. I thanked God for this lifeline, a chance to continue my journey, and a purpose to my existence.

In the year that followed my arrival in Hawaii, I prepared diligently for the proposed brain surgery. The gamma knife brain surgery, known as stereotactic radiosurgery, was on the horizon, and it demanded my utmost readiness. Daily, I pushed myself, engaging in runs and weightlifting, determined to be in the best possible condition for the impending procedure. Each day was a testament to my will to survive to make the most of the second chance that had been granted to me.

As the day of the surgery arrived, all pre-operative preparations were meticulously completed. I stepped into the hospital, ready to face the daunting gamma knife, a powerful tool in the battle against my brain tumor. However, what transpired next was a startling twist that I had not foreseen.

In the surgical theater, my brilliant doctor engaged in a heated, loud exchange with the attending physician. Their voices rose in a crescendo of emotions, and it soon became clear that they were locked in a passionate disagreement. My doctor was fervently pleading with the attending physician, expressing his fear that the surgery would prove fatal. Somehow, meeting me in person had overwhelmed him with emotion, and he was now battling to save my life.

Summoning every ounce of strength within me, I raised my voice, demanding that the heated argument between my two doctors cease immediately. The gravity of the situation was palpable, but I was determined not to let chaos interfere with the procedure that would determine my fate. My resolve was unwavering, and as I lay on the surgical table, I planned to document the entire event. The thought of a video diary entry crossed my mind, a testament to the fact that I had never given up on the quest to save my own life.

As the doctors continued their exchange, I remained remarkably calm. Deep within, I felt a sense of confidence and serenity, a belief that a higher power was guiding the course of events. It was God who held the reins, and my faith assured me that everything would unfold as it should. Against all odds, I was still alive, defying the expectations that had once cast a dark shadow over my future.

In a moment of quiet reflection, I offered a prayer, a plea for strength and protection during the trial that lay ahead. The "crown of thorns," as I saw it, was a symbol of the divine shield that would guard me in my moment of need. I was, after all, one of God's children, and I knew that His watchful eye would oversee the events that would soon transpire.

My doctor began the procedure by meticulously securing a metal frame into my head. This simple yet crucial step was necessary to ensure that I would remain immobile during the radiation therapy. The frame would be attached to the radiation table, allowing the super-concentrated beams of radiation to target the precise spot where the tumor lurked. The stakes were high, and precision was paramount in this complex and delicate process.

As the radiation beams were delivered, I lay there, still and resolute, feeling the tension in the room gradually dissipate. I was eventually unscrewed from the table, and the metal frame was removed from my head. The procedure was completed without incident, leaving me with a profound sense of relief. This was just another medical appointment on my journey, accompanied by fervent prayer and, miraculously, no complications.

This form of radiation therapy, known as stereotactic radiosurgery, was primarily employed to treat brain tumors. It wasn't my first encounter with radiation therapy, and I couldn't help but wonder how much more my body could withstand. Yet, in the midst of my thoughts, a comforting reminder emerged – this was a far safer alternative to traditional brain surgery, a fact that provided me with a degree of solace.

The procedure, I was informed, might be mildly uncomfortable, and there were moments when it would cause pain. Nevertheless, everything went remarkably well, exceeding expectations. The team of doctors wore pleased expressions, and my own doctor's confidence had proven to be well-founded.

Returning home after the procedure, I found myself burdened by an intense, burning headache. The brain swelling had surged with a relentless force, making its presence known almost immediately. It was back to the familiar routine of dexamethasone, the corticosteroid drug that had become my companion in this harrowing journey. Dexamethasone's role was clear – to combat inflammation by taming the body's immune response. For over a year, I had relied on this medication, with each dose being stronger and longer-lasting than the last. It had been my lifeline, a temporary respite from the relentless swelling in my brain.

However, my solace would be short-lived. Four months down the road, I found myself hospitalized, the victim of severe brain swelling that had emerged as a side effect of the radiation surgery. The once-effective treatment now seemed to falter, and the future appeared shrouded in uncertainty. It was a disheartening moment, and the flicker of hope that had sustained me through the darkest days of my journey was now dimming.

As I lay in that hospital bed, the most worrisome hospital visit to date, my faith was tested. The questions that had lingered on the fringes of my mind now clawed their way to the forefront. Had I come this far only to face the grim specter of death? Doubt crept in, but I remained steadfast in my resolve. I could not, and would not, surrender. I told myself that I was still far too stubborn, too determined, too mean to die.

In my darkest hour, when hope seemed to dwindle, divine intervention arrived in the form of a new neurosurgeon. He entered my life as an angel on Earth, bearing the message that would chart the course of my survival. With a reassuring demeanor, he presented the solution that would save my life – Avastin.

Avastin was an immunotherapy agent, a beacon of hope that promised to "calm down" the damage caused by radiation and halt the relentless brain swelling. It was the lifeline I had been waiting for, a remedy that could potentially alter the course of my battle. It was as if God, in His infinite wisdom, had sent this physician to deliver the final message, the key to my continued existence.

After spending eight seemingly endless days in the hospital, I was finally released and swiftly ushered into the next phase of my treatment journey. My new oncologist had charted a course for me, one that involved a series of four planned Avastin treatments to be administered intravenously. It was a pivotal juncture, and I was cautiously optimistic about the road that lay ahead. To my astonishment, I had miraculously avoided the need for a port, and my veins, which had endured the rigors of previous chemotherapy treatments, had completely healed.

As I settled into the rhythm of the Avastin treatments, I was soon to realize that the real battle was only just beginning. After my very first intravenous infusion of Avastin, my body reacted strongly, and I found myself grappling with severe side effects. It was a daunting start to a treatment that held so much promise. The treatment plan called for these immunotherapy infusions every two weeks, and I was slated to endure eight weeks of this rigorous regimen.

Avastin, as it turned out, posed not only a medical challenge but a financial one as well. The staggering cost of each dose, nearly $18,000, loomed like a shadow over my hopes. I was faced with the arduous task of convincing my insurance to cover this vital treatment. It seemed like an insurmountable hurdle, but once again, fate would shine upon me. My insurance agreed to cover the expenses with one small caveat – a $750 copay was due at each infusion. Overwhelmed by the financial burden, I was relieved when my compassionate oncologist allowed me to make payments. It was a debt I was willing to shoulder if it meant the chance to continue fighting for my life.

My body, however, had its own limits, and it became evident that after six weeks of treatments, I could endure no more. Severe gastrointestinal distress took hold, causing excruciating pain and pushing me to the brink of another hospitalization. It was a moment of surrender, a recognition that my fatigued body had reached its threshold. I made the difficult decision to halt the Avastin treatments and ventured into the unknown, not knowing what lay ahead.

So, what did happen next? Brace yourself because the twists and turns of this journey were far from over, and the story that unfolded was one that seemed almost unbelievable.

Throughout this tumultuous journey, one thing remained steadfast – my unwavering faith. I had made a solemn vow to myself and to God on that fateful day of my Gamma Knife surgery, July 10, 2014. It was a promise that no matter how trying the path might become, I would emerge victorious. As I put these words down on paper, I am on the cusp of celebrating my ten-year anniversary since that life-altering radio-brain surgery. It's a milestone that fills me with profound gratitude and awe, for I stand here today, a living testament to the power of faith and the resilience of the human spirit.

Incredibly, I now bear no evidence of the brain tumor that once loomed as a daunting specter in my life. None. The same holds true for my battle with breast cancer – no evidence remains. It's a reality that often leaves me in awe, prompting questions that defy easy answers. How could it be possible that I not only survived but triumphed over two nearly fatal diagnoses? What set my journey apart from the countless others who face the same trials? The answer, I believe, lies in the potent combination of prayer and unwavering faith.

Leaning into my beliefs and placing my trust in a higher power was the compass that guided me through the darkest days. It was a journey that defied the odds, a testament to the remarkable strides made by modern medicine and the immeasurable power of prayer. The synergy of the two was the alchemy that turned despair into hope and adversity into triumph.

Is the power of prayer the constant, unwavering energy that rescues us when all seems lost? In my heart and soul, the answer resounds with a resounding "yes." I was never alone on this arduous path, for God was with me every step of the way, carrying me through the trials and tribulations. It's why, as I look back, there's only one set of footprints in the sand.

Psalm 77:19 - Your path led through the sea, your way through the mighty waters, though your footprints were not seen.

What have I learned from this chapter?

CHAPTER 7
EMOTIONAL CLUTTER

Life after breast cancer and a brain tumor diagnosis is a profound testament to the incredible strength, unwavering resilience, and indomitable determination that resided within me, waiting to be unveiled. It's a chapter of my life that showcases the incredible power of the human spirit to not just survive but to thrive.

When confronted with the harrowing reality of my illnesses, I found solace in faith. I reached out to God, seeking the strength to face these formidable adversaries, and miraculously, I received it. With newfound determination, I embarked on a journey of rediscovery. This was my chance to uncover the dormant layers of my identity, to explore the boundless reservoirs of joy that life had to offer.

My decision to share my battle with cancer is born out of gratitude. Gratitude for the very breath that sustains me, for the chance to embrace life with a new perspective, and for the privilege to stand as a beacon of hope for others. It's a testament to the enduring human spirit, which, when met with adversity, can shine brighter and more resilient than ever before.

As I sit here, the arduous path of my breast cancer and brain tumor treatment journey has come to a close. Yet, as one chapter closes, many others swing wide open. It's a journey of self-discovery that continuously unfolds, bringing new experiences and opportunities, not only for me but for you as well.

Life post-cancer is about finding joy in the smallest of moments. It's about navigating through the emotional clutter that remains after the storm. It's about adapting to the 'new normal,' where scars are badges of honor and reminders of the battles won.

Every milestone, from the completion of treatments to the first follow-up appointment, is a significant victory over the shadows of cancer. Each step forward is a reason for celebration, a testament to the remarkable resilience of the human body and spirit.

Above all, this post-cancer life is a journey to be lived with gratitude. Gratitude for the gift of each day, for the opportunity to see the world through different eyes, and for the chance to share my story with you. Life is a beautiful and unpredictable journey, and I intend to savor every moment of it.

The journey post-treatment is a challenging path for survivors, one that demands acknowledgment of their incredible achievements and the pursuit of joy in the progress they've made. After the last treatment, the cancer was defeated, and I had hoped to effortlessly bounce back to the life I had known before cancer entered my world. Yet, the reality was quite different.

It was, in fact, post-treatment where the most arduous battle began. The physical changes and challenges were not to be underestimated. This, I discovered, was perhaps the most difficult part of the entire journey. I had to relearn the art of being gentle with myself. The cancer was gone, but I was left with a body and mind that bore the scars of the struggle. It was a sobering realization, and I had to manage my own expectations to truly embark on the path of healing.

To heal, I first had to accept myself. It was a profound lesson. My body needed time to recover, and it demanded patience and understanding. The post-cancer journey was a metamorphosis, not a return to the past. I found myself gradually rebuilding, relearning, and reshaping my perception of self. I had to learn to love this new version of my mind and body.

Yet, I wished someone had prepared me for the challenges that lay beyond treatment. I was startled by the changes in my body – the asymmetry, the new scars that told a story of battles fought and won. I grappled with my reflection, and there were moments when I felt like I had lost the battle. It was then that I'd joke with myself, reminding me that my body, with the aid of treatment, had bravely vanquished the tumor.

The post-cancer journey was, and still is, a process of self-acceptance, of understanding that my body was a battlefield where strength and courage had triumphed. It's a journey of resilience, where each scar tells a story of survival. As I continue to move forward, I carry these scars as badges of honor, and I'm learning to love the person I've become – a survivor, filled with gratitude for the gift of each new day.

As I journeyed my way through the labyrinth of breast cancer treatment, I found myself standing at a crossroads, facing a myriad of surgical options. Each choice was influenced by a delicate interplay of factors, such as the stage of my cancer, the tumor's size and location, and my own personal preferences. These decisions were pivotal in shaping my path towards recovery.

One of the options that lay before me was the lumpectomy, also known as breast-conserving surgery. This procedure offered a glimmer of hope, involving the removal of the tumor and a small margin of surrounding healthy tissue while preserving my breast. It was a path filled with promise, one that often led to radiation therapy, but it allowed me to hold onto a part of myself.

On the other side of the spectrum was the mastectomy, a surgical route that necessitated the removal of the entire breast. It was a more radical choice, but sometimes it was the only way forward. Mastectomy, I learned, had its own variations, including the simple or total mastectomy, which preserved the lymph nodes and underlying muscle tissue. Then, there was the modified radical mastectomy, which involved excising both the breast and some lymph nodes. Lastly, the rarely performed radical mastectomy went even further, removing not just the breast but also the chest muscles and lymph nodes from the armpit.

The journey did not end there. In my quest to understand the extent of cancer's reach, I encountered the sentinel lymph node biopsy, a procedure that aimed to identify and remove the most likely nodes to harbor cancer cells, providing insight into whether the cancer had ventured into the lymphatic system. For those situations where cancer had ventured further, the axillary lymph node dissection became a necessity, as the surgeon removed additional lymph nodes from the armpit area to ensure comprehensive treatment.

Amidst these decisions, the notion of breast reconstruction emerged as an optional yet profound choice. It was an opportunity to rebuild not just the physical aspect of my body but also the emotional one. Whether performed alongside mastectomy or as a separate surgery, it aimed to restore the appearance and shape of my breast through various methods like implants, tissue expanders, or autologous tissue reconstruction, often referred to as a "flap" reconstruction.

In the midst of this intricate tapestry of decisions, I came to realize the significance of seeking counsel from a proficient healthcare team, comprising a committed breast surgeon and oncologist. Their expertise empowered them to assess my individual circumstances and provide tailor-made advice, thus guiding me towards the surgical option most suited to my breast cancer treatment. It was a voyage through a spectrum of choices, with each one assuming a crucial role in my fight against cancer and my pursuit of a healthier future.

As I had previously shared in an earlier chapter, my breast cancer journey has been a complex one, punctuated by a series of two lumpectomies on my left breast since my initial diagnosis in 2011. However, the year 2017 brought its own set of challenges. I found myself undergoing three lumpectomies on my right breast, as there were suspicious masses that, according to the laboratory findings, turned out to be precancerous lesions. Additionally, I had to go through the procedure of having my sentinel lymph node removed on my left side, marking another step in my ongoing battle with cancer.

Life after cancer is a profound transformation. I knew I had to regain my strength and sanity. To accomplish this, I embarked on a journey of rebuilding both my mind and body. Regular exercise, a balanced diet, and the commitment to a healthy lifestyle became my allies in the quest to reclaim my vitality.

Regaining my former fitness seemed like an insurmountable challenge. When I attempted to run after chemotherapy and radiation treatment, it was a humbling experience. I barely took a few steps before feeling nauseous, eventually leading to an unfortunate bout of vomiting. What I once took for granted now felt like an ascent up an imaginary mountain. That first attempt ended with me in tears, and my hair coated in vomit. I was shaken to my core, but I refused to give up.

This experience led me to question God once more. Why was I chosen to survive only to endure such misery? Would it always be this arduous, this painful? The bone pain and neuropathy that lingered after Taxol treatment were harsh realities. Regrettably, they have become permanent side effects. I've learned to manage the deep bone pain with the soothing touch of heat and massages. In moments of acute discomfort, topical lidocaine patches, readily available at every drugstore, have offered a measure of relief.

Through these trials and tribulations, I found a tenacious spirit within myself. The journey through cancer is filled with unexpected challenges, but it's also a testament to the human capacity for resilience and determination. I keep pushing forward, one step at a time, in the pursuit of a healthier and more vibrant tomorrow.

That day, I never received a direct answer from God. Instead, I found myself overwhelmed by a sense of defeat, tears marking my path as I cried myself to sleep. It was moments like these that spurred me to write this book, to share my experiences and let you know that it does get better. The journey won't always be this difficult; I pinky swear on it. You must remember to surrender your worries to God, allowing the feelings of loss and sorrow to dissipate. It's okay to mourn the person you once were, but you must also learn to celebrate your rebirth, like a phoenix rising from the ashes.

Along the path to recovery, embrace the support available from healthcare professionals, including acupuncturists, physical therapists, and nutritionists. Their expertise can offer guidance and further assist in your physical recovery. Discover what makes you feel well again, for nutrition plays a crucial role in a speedy recovery. Keep a vigilant eye on your Vitamin D levels, as there is a clear connection between Vitamin D and cancer. Maintaining your levels above 50 is a proactive step in preventing a reoccurrence. Studies have illuminated the link between vitamin D levels and overall health; it's a lesson I learned the hard way when my own levels plummeted just before my initial diagnosis.

But it's not just about the physical healing; your emotional well-being is equally important. The emotional impact of breast cancer can be profound, with lingering feelings of fear, anxiety, and uncertainty that persist even after treatment concludes. A very real phenomenon known as "scanxiety" can grip you during routine aftercare CT or

PET scans. Coined by cancer survivors, scanxiety encapsulates the anxiety that can consume you as you await the results of these vital tests. While treatment may be over, the lifetime of monitoring is just beginning. Learning the lingo and navigating the emotional terrain is a significant part of the healing journey.

In the chapters of my medical journey, the CT scan, or computed tomography scan, emerged as a crucial player. It's a remarkable medical imaging procedure, a bit like a high-tech detective story, allowing a detailed look inside the intricate landscapes of the human body. The CT scan wields a combination of X-rays and computer technology to create cross-sectional images that reveal the hidden mysteries within.

In the course of a CT scan, I would recline upon a table that gracefully traversed through a ring-shaped apparatus known as a CT scanner. This advanced machine would emit a sequence of X-ray beams from various angles encircling my body. Inside the machine, detectors meticulously gauged the radiation's passage through my body. Subsequently, this intricately collected data would be methodically processed by a computer, giving rise to an array of meticulous images or cross-sectional slices dedicated to the specific area under examination.

CT scans are like magic windows for doctors, offering a more comprehensive view of internal structures. They unveil the secrets of our organs, bones, blood vessels, and soft tissues with stunning clarity. These scans have revolutionized the world of medical diagnostics, surpassing the capabilities of traditional X-rays.

The scope of what a CT scan can achieve is truly awe-inspiring. It's a versatile tool that can help identify and assess various conditions, from injuries and infections to tumors, cardiovascular diseases, and anomalies lurking in the brain or other organs. But its powers extend beyond mere diagnosis; CT scans are also instrumental in guiding medical procedures, such as biopsies or planning for radiation therapy.

However, it's essential to remember that every coin has two sides. CT scans, while incredibly valuable, come with a cautionary note. They involve exposure to ionizing radiation, a potential risk that must be weighed against the benefits they offer. This duality makes every journey through the CT scanner a calculated decision, where the quest for knowledge meets the need for caution.

Within the pages of my medical journey, the PET scan emerged as another essential tool in the quest for understanding my health. It's a fascinating medical imaging technique that delves beyond mere structure, providing a window into the metabolic activity of the body. Unlike conventional imaging methods like X-rays or CT scans, PET scans offer a glimpse into the dynamic function and vitality of tissues and organs.

During a PET scan, I would find myself in a dimly lit room, where a small amount of a radioactive tracer, known as a radiopharmaceutical, was gently injected into my vein.

This tracer was often designed to mimic substances like glucose or oxygen – compounds that cells in the body metabolize as part of their natural processes. What makes these tracers remarkable is that they're tagged with a radioactive isotope that emits positrons and positively charged particles.

As this radiopharmaceutical coursed through my body, it was absorbed by different tissues and organs in varying amounts, reflecting their metabolic activity. The positrons emitted by the tracer engaged with electrons in my body, giving rise to gamma rays. Sensitive detectors within the PET scanner captured these gamma rays, crafting intricate three-dimensional images that painted a vivid picture of areas exhibiting high metabolic activity.

The significance of PET scans in the realm of oncology cannot be overstated. Their ability to detect and assess cancer is invaluable. Cancer cells tend to possess higher metabolic rates than their normal counterparts, rendering them regions with heightened tracer uptake on the PET scan. This critical information aids in the staging of cancer, gauging the extent of its spread, and monitoring the response to treatment.

But PET scans aren't confined to oncology. They're versatile detectives in the world of medicine, employed to diagnose and assess a range of conditions. From probing into heart disease and delving into the intricacies of brain disorders like Alzheimer's disease to investigating certain types of infections, PET scans offer a holistic view of the body's physiology, complementing other imaging tests like CT or MRI scans.

It's vital to acknowledge that PET scans do involve exposure to radiation due to the use of radioactive tracers. However, these doses are carefully controlled and considered safe, with the diagnostic benefits far outweighing the potential risks. The procedure is executed under vigilant supervision, with radiation exposure minimized to the extent reasonably achievable.

The message embedded in this journey is clear: knowledge is power. And as I've learned, it's also crucial to prepare for the reality of post-cancer aftercare. For the initial years following treatment, my doctor maintained a close watch for any hints of recurrence. These are the moments when it becomes essential to find joy within oneself, celebrating the strength, resilience, and unwavering spirit that has carried us through the storm.

Embracing the journey of post-cancer recovery comes with its unique set of challenges, and it's not limited to the physical aspect alone. Prioritizing emotional well-being is just as crucial during this phase. It's a time to acknowledge that healing encompasses more than just the mending of the body; it involves nurturing the spirit and mind.

Support groups, self-help books, therapy, or counseling sessions can become sanctuaries for the expression of emotions, the sharing of experiences, and the connection with others who have trod similar paths. I discovered that these safe spaces allowed me to articulate my innermost thoughts and fears, offering solace in the knowledge that I wasn't alone in my journey.

Another avenue for healing was engaging in self-care activities. Meditation, yoga, writing, or exploring new hobbies became beacons of hope on the road to emotional recovery. It was a time to indulge in whatever made me feel better because there's no one-size-fits-all approach to healing. It's vital to recognize that recovery often involves accepting the highs and lows, granting oneself the grace to take a break from the arduous process when needed. After all, healing isn't bound by time or deadlines. The journey can't be rushed or pressured. It unfolds at its own pace, unique to each survivor.

Breast cancer and its treatments can significantly alter a survivor's body image and self-esteem. Adjusting to the changes post-cancer, whether it's mastectomy scars or hair loss, can be an uphill battle. However, it's essential to grasp that true beauty emanates from within and manifests in diverse forms. Our self-worth stretches far beyond our physical appearance.

Support is a lifeline in this journey. Loved ones, support groups, and resources like tattoos, prosthetics, and reconstructive surgery can play pivotal roles in rebuilding confidence and embracing one's body anew. The advances in the modern age are truly astounding.

For instance, I chose to tattoo over my scars with ink that perfectly matched my skin tone, making them less conspicuous. Paramedical tattoos have become a popular solution for permanent scar cover-up. Experts in the field can now create 3-D areolas and nipples, offering survivors a chance to reclaim their sense of self. Some even opt for lace bra tattoos over mastectomy scars, their options boundless.

Reconstructive surgery is another avenue to explore fully. Engaging with fellow survivors can provide invaluable insights and feedback, offering a clearer perspective on the choices available.

Within the chapters of my breast cancer journey, the path to breast reconstruction post-lumpectomies became a significant milestone. It's a deeply personal decision, one influenced by an array of factors, including my own anatomy, overall health, and, of course, personal preferences. I encountered a realm of options, each with its unique characteristics.

One common route is implant-based reconstruction, which involves using breast implants to recreate the shape and size of the breast. This journey typically unfolds in two stages. In the initial surgery, a tissue expander, essentially an inflatable implant, is placed to gradually stretch the skin and chest muscles. Subsequent surgeries follow, wherein the tissue expander is replaced with a permanent implant, bringing the reconstruction to its conclusion.

Then there's the path of autologous tissue (flap) reconstruction, where a survivor's own tissue, usually sourced from the abdomen, back, or buttocks, serves as the raw material for breast reconstruction. Here, a variety of techniques come into play:

- TRAM flap (transverse rectus abdominis muscle): This method utilizes muscle, fat, and skin from the lower abdomen to craft a new breast mound.
- DIEP flap (deep inferior epigastric perforator): Similar to the TRAM flap but with a notable difference – it preserves the abdominal muscles, utilizing solely the skin and fat for the reconstruction process.
- Latissimus dorsi flap: In this approach, muscle, fat, and skin from the upper back are brought under the skin to the chest, forming a new breast shape. This method might necessitate an implant for added volume.

However, life is not always lived in black and white. There's also the option of combination or hybrid reconstruction, where a blend of implant-based and autologous tissue reconstruction is employed to achieve the desired outcome. This path allows for greater flexibility in crafting the breast, as it melds the benefits of both approaches.

The selection of a breast reconstruction method is a deeply personal one. It's an intricate puzzle where factors like overall health, body shape, available donor sites, and individual preferences come together. In my own journey, I found it invaluable to engage in detailed discussions with a plastic surgeon specializing in breast reconstruction. This expert can offer insights into the benefits, potential risks, and expected outcomes of each technique, tailored to my specific circumstances.

The decision to forego reconstructive breast surgery after my partial mastectomy was a deeply personal one and I've found peace and contentment with that choice. In this journey, I've come to understand the profound importance of doing what feels right for oneself and seeking happiness on one's own terms. It's about focusing on the present and embracing who I've become after the battle with cancer.

Regular follow-up appointments and screenings have become a vital part of my post-treatment life. These ongoing check-ins and early detection measures are essential for ensuring that any potential recurrence is swiftly identified and addressed. Staying proactive about healthcare and maintaining open lines of communication with my medical professionals have been pivotal in this ongoing battle. Survivorship care plans have provided valuable guidance on post-treatment care, recommending necessary screenings, suggesting lifestyle adjustments, and helping manage the long-term effects of treatment.

Breast cancer has a way of reshaping a survivor's perspective on life. It often leads to a quest for deeper meaning and purpose, prompting a newfound appreciation for the precious gift of life. I, too, cherish my life now more than ever. At times, I find myself pondering what would have been missed had I given up the fight. A decade of milestones, the joy of meeting my beautiful grandchild, Cassie, the fulfillment of writing this very book, and the pursuit of meaningful goals – these are the treasures I've uncovered in my post-cancer life. My journey has transformed me into a joyful warrior, and it's a path that's open to anyone.

Breast cancer survivors possess a unique opportunity to become advocates and mentors for those facing similar challenges. Sharing our personal stories, raising awareness, and supporting initiatives focused on early detection and research can have a profound impact. Engaging with local or online support communities allows survivors to extend their hand in support and guidance, fostering empowerment and reinforcing the idea that we are never alone. We are pink sisters, bound by an unchosen membership, but one that we can make the best of.

Life after breast cancer stands as a testament to the strength, resilience, and unwavering determination of all survivors. It's a poignant reminder that each one of us is surviving something painful in our own history. By embracing the journey and extending our support to one another, survivors can navigate this new chapter with hope, courage, and a renewed appreciation for the precious gift of life. In these moments, I am reminded that God never makes mistakes, and this new path is guiding me closer to my destiny.

After the long and challenging journey through cancer and a brain tumor, the path to recovery was multifaceted. It encompassed not only emotional and physical healing but also the daunting task of addressing the negative financial impact that cancer can have on one's life. Recovering financially from the rigors of treatment is a journey of its own, and while it's no easy road, there are strategies that can help.

One crucial step is to review your health insurance coverage. It's vital to understand your policy and benefits so you can discern which costs are covered and which expenses you'll need to manage. Look out for deductibles, co-pays, or out-of-pocket maximums, as these will play a significant role in your financial planning.

In this endeavor, it's important not to let pride stand in the way. There are assistance programs available, and there's no shame in applying for them. I wholeheartedly encourage seeking out government programs, nonprofit organizations, and foundations that offer financial assistance for cancer patients. These avenues can extend a helping hand with medication costs, transportation, housing, and other financial burdens.

Communication with your healthcare providers is equally essential. Don't hesitate to share your financial concerns with your healthcare team. They may have insights into cost-saving measures, be able to connect you with discounted medications or refer you to financial counselors who specialize in managing medical bills. If the situation calls for it, consider seeking financial counseling to create a budget, negotiate medical bills, explore payment plans, or even apply for medical debt forgiveness programs.

Moreover, researching local resources can lead to valuable support. Many support groups, community organizations, or cancer centers offer financial assistance, counseling, or workshops on managing medical expenses. It's a reservoir of knowledge and help waiting to be tapped into.

Exploring crowdfunding platforms like GoFundMe is another way to address financial challenges. Setting up a crowdfunding campaign can provide an opportunity to receive support from friends, family, or even compassionate strangers who are willing to contribute to your medical expenses.

Never undcrestimate the power of asking for help, and remember that there's no shame in doing so. Cancer and its aftermath are formidable challenges, and it's a journey that's meant to be shared.

As for me, I embarked on a complete life rebuild after surviving cancer and a brain tumor. I vividly recall the time when I was fighting for my life and gave away my possessions. The panic was real, but I took it one day at a time. In rebuilding my life, I felt as though I had been reborn. I didn't grieve for the material possessions I had given away; instead, I embraced the adventure of rebuilding not only my health but also my home and financial well-being. The Phoenix had indeed risen from the ashes.

Today, I find myself in a place of abundance and joy that I never dreamed of having again. Life remains beautiful because I am alive and thriving. God has blessed me with more than I could have imagined.

Sometimes, I forget I ever had cancer because every day is filled with joy. I've filled my life with so much happiness that the pain and sadness have become distant memories.

In the journey of recovery, you, too, will become immersed in your post-cancer life, and the pain will fade into the background as you reframe your life with happiness.

CHAPTER 8
THE POWER OF COLLECTIVE ENERGY AND HEALING

The incredible power of collective energy and healing played a significant role in my cancer journey. It's the idea that when individuals unite with a shared intention or focus, their combined energy can create a powerful force that amplifies and enhances the healing process. This collective energy goes beyond the individual and encompasses physical, emotional, and even spiritual healing.

During my cancer treatment, the importance of a supportive and uplifting environment became evident. It's the very foundation that allowed me to successfully navigate the challenging path of treatment. This collective energy nurtured a sense of unity, empathy, and connection among us, which, in turn, contributed to a deeper and more meaningful healing experience.

I've come to realize that the impact of collective healing extends far beyond the individual. It can likely alter entire communities, promoting well-being and positive change. It's a reminder that we don't have to face these challenges alone.

In my own journey, I've learned the profound value of asking for help and seeking prayers, even when I wasn't entirely sure what I needed. It's a way of allowing your community to find you and support you. The collective prayers and intentions from your community can be a source of unbelievable strength and healing.

What is a prayer, and how can it help me?

A prayer is a form of communication or expression that is directed towards a higher power or deity. It is a way of respectfully making requests, offering thanks, or expressing one's supplication, often through words or in a ritualistic manner. Prayers take various forms across different religions and cultures, but their common purpose is to seek guidance, solace, or a connection with the divine.

My own journey through life has exposed me to different religions and belief systems. I was baptized Catholic at birth, but my mother's hardships led me to be embraced by other families with varying cultural and religious backgrounds. This experience opened my eyes to the common thread that unites people from different walks of life – the belief in a higher power.

During my cancer journey, seeking guidance, solace, and connection became vital, in my opinion. I've previously mentioned the importance of giving your worries back to God. It's about allowing God to shoulder the burdens that become too heavy to bear on your own. This, I believe, is a common thread that not only helps individuals survive cancer but also provides strength in overcoming various other life challenges.

Prayer is a powerful source of comfort, solace, and a profound sense of connection for many individuals. It provides a sacred space for self-reflection, expressing gratitude, seeking guidance, and finding inner strength. It's a practice that fosters a deep sense of community and shared values among those who come together in prayer.

Imagine people from all corners of the world collectively uttering your name and beseeching the divine for healing. The energy and support transferred through such collective prayers are real. During my own treatment, I reached out and asked for prayers from everyone, and it became a profound source of comfort, knowing that countless individuals were invoking my name to reach God's ear, seeking healing on my behalf. I firmly believe that God heard those prayers and played a pivotal role in my recovery. It defies rational explanation; the medical treatment alone couldn't account for my survival, especially in the face of near-fatal adverse reactions.

For some, prayer is a profound way to find inner peace and meaning and to nurture a deeper spiritual connection. It's essential to acknowledge that the impact of prayer can vary among individuals with differing religious beliefs, but the underlying positive emotions remain the same.

During my own challenging times, certain Bible verses provided me with immense comfort and strength. These verses were like guiding beacons, illuminating the path through the darkest moments in my life. They served as a source of hope and resilience, reminding me that there was a higher power guiding me through the storm.

Jeremiah 30:17 - "But I restore you to health and heal your wounds, declares the Lord." These words, spoken with unwavering belief, were like a sacred incantation. I asked for restoration, for healing, and miraculously, my health was indeed restored, and my wounds were healed. Over time, even most of my scars have faded, a testament to the miraculous healing that has taken place in my body.

Psalm 6:2 - "Have mercy on me, Lord, for I am faint. Heal me, Lord, for my bones are in agony." During the grueling Taxol treatment, when bone pain threatened to overwhelm me, I clung to this verse. I beseeched for mercy, and mercy was granted. It became my lifeline, helping me persevere through the darkest hours, even when hope seemed scarce.

Psalm 34:18 - "The Lord is close to the brokenhearted and saves those who are crushed in spirit." Cancer has a way of breaking one's spirit, but these words reminded me that I was never truly alone. It was as if the verse was whispered directly to me, offering reassurance that God would be my savior, no matter the adversity.

Wisdom of Solomon 16:12 - "It wasn't any herb or ointment that healed them but your word alone, Lord, which heals everything." These words highlight the immense power of God's word in bringing about healing. Speaking the words of the Lord, I experienced their profound impact on my reality, guiding me toward recovery and wellness.

Did my prayers ultimately save my life and heal me? While we can never be entirely certain, I stand as a living testament to the miraculous power of faith. I have been healed with no evidence of cancer or a brain tumor. I am a living miracle, and my story is shared with the hope of inspiring others facing similar challenges.

Lastly, *Psalm 41:3 assures that "The Lord sustains them on their sickbed and restores them from their bed of illness."* These words have provided unwavering comfort, reminding me that God's sustenance and restoration are ever-present, even in the darkest moments of illness.

Life after cancer is a testament to resilience, healing, and the pursuit of dreams. The battle against this devastating disease is one that should never be underestimated. Cancer's impact, both physical and emotional, is immense, leaving individuals feeling shattered and bereft of joy. Yet, even in the midst of darkness, it's possible to rediscover joy and purpose. I've experienced this transformation firsthand and wish to inspire you to embrace a joyful life, even in times of hardship.

The journey to joy begins with acknowledging and understanding the profound emotional impact of cancer. This disease often unleashes a tidal wave of emotions, including fear, grief, and anxiety. By allowing these emotions to surface and working through them, survivors can pave the way for joy to reenter their lives.

A positive mindset is an essential companion on the path to joy after cancer. It involves cultivating gratitude, living in the present moment, and transforming negative thoughts. For me, I've made a conscious choice never to revisit negative thoughts. When they threaten to resurface, I redirect my focus to more positive views and activities. It takes practice, but eventually, it becomes a natural response when darker memories attempt to intrude.

The message is clear - Cancer survivors can find joy, a renewed sense of purpose, and a brighter outlook on life. Survivors who adopt a positive outlook often discover the strength to overcome challenges and embrace life's many offerings. One of the key pillars supporting this transformation is a strong support network. Personally, I owe immeasurable gratitude to each person who played a part in my cancer journey. Words alone can never fully express my appreciation for the boundless kindness and generosity that myself and my family received during those challenging times. For the past decade, I've dedicated myself to expressing my gratitude and repaying those who stood by us.

The gift of connecting with fellow survivors, friends, family, and support groups was a lifeline for me. Sharing stories and experiences with others who've traversed similar paths empowers us and contributes to the rediscovery of joy after cancer.

Cancer often prompts a profound reevaluation of priorities, leading us to unearth new sources of meaning and purpose. In my own life post-cancer, I've uncovered a completely fresh sense of purpose. This includes sharing my miraculous story with others. Equally important, it's been a mission of mine to reclaim the precious time that cancer had tried to steal from my family and me. Being the best grandmother I can be to my darling granddaughter, Miss Cassie Brooke, has become a primary focus.

I am profoundly thankful that I never gave up. It's a message I'd like to convey to you as well. I cheer you to embark on a journey of self-discovery, seeking activities and passions that ignite your joy and fulfillment.

Engaging in cherished hobbies and creative pursuits can rekindle your sense of purpose and infuse daily life with joy. Physical well-being, I've discovered, is intrinsically linked to emotional well-being. My daily walks energize me and provide moments of clarity. The adoption of a healthy lifestyle—complete with regular exercise, a balanced diet, and ample rest—contributes significantly to the overall well-being of cancer survivors.

It's essential to take charge of your health and well-being and find ways to make the most of your post-cancer life. Sometimes, a simple step in a new direction, like signing up for a half marathon, can lead to an empowered and happier you. It's not about finishing the marathon but about taking the courageous step to start, knowing that the journey itself is a victory.

Physical activities hold the power to elevate your mood, diminish stress, and invigorate your energy levels, creating a more fertile ground for joy to flourish. Mindfulness and self-care are the cornerstones of rediscovering yourself and finding joy after the arduous battle with cancer. Mindful practices like meditation and deep breathing exercises serve as anchors, grounding survivors in the present moment, assisting them in stress management, and revealing the beauty surrounding them.

Self-care practices are a sanctuary for moments of joy and revitalization. Pampering oneself, diving into beloved hobbies, or immersing in nature's embrace can be a wellspring of happiness. Amid this journey, one significant aspect is acknowledging and celebrating milestones and victories, no matter how small they may seem. Survivors can mark the anniversaries of their journey, significant treatment milestones, or personal accomplishments, letting these moments serve as reflections of their remarkable strength and resilience. It is in these milestones that they can find the joy in their progress, the joy in their survival.

Finding joy after cancer is a profoundly personal and transformative journey. It encompasses a variety of steps - acknowledging the emotional impact, fostering a positive mindset, building a supportive network, unearthing meaning and purpose, nurturing physical well-being, embracing mindfulness and self-care, and commemorating milestones. Each of these steps might pose its own challenges, but it's within these challenges that the strength, resilience, and unique ability to find joy, even in the face of adversity, shine through. You are, without a doubt, stronger than you might know. Live joyfully, for you have earned it, and become a true joyful warrior, triumphing over adversity.

The final leg of my healing journey was a profound exploration of forgiveness, a process that allowed me to release the weight of sadness and resentment lingering in my life, particularly concerning my mother and my battle with cancer. Letting go of pain and offering forgiveness, I discovered, can be even more challenging than facing cancer head-on. But, when you genuinely forgive someone, it's like unlocking a door to newfound freedom.

The act of forgiving individuals who have caused you harm or heartache yields numerous benefits for your overall well-being and healing process. Let me share some of these invaluable benefits.

First and foremost, forgiveness unshackles you from the heavy burden of anger, resentment, and bitterness. It's like casting off an anchor that has been weighing you down for far too long. This newfound lightness allows you to let go of negative emotions and reclaim your emotional well-being. By relinquishing the grip of these detrimental feelings, forgiveness creates ample space for healing and the emergence of positive emotions.

Joy and positivity played a pivotal role in my life as I ventured through the labyrinth of post-cancer existence. Their interconnection is profound and symbiotic, exerting a tremendous influence on our overall well-being and the quality of our lives.

Positivity acts as a powerful catalyst for experiencing joy. When we adopt a positive outlook, we tend to view situations through a lens of optimism, focusing on the potential for growth, learning, and happiness. This optimistic perspective opens our hearts and minds to the vast realm of joy, allowing us to recognize and appreciate the positive facets of our lives.

Positivity doesn't merely influence our outlook; it directly impacts our emotional state. It creates an environment conducive to experiencing joy. By maintaining a positive mindset, we're more likely to feel uplifted, content, and grateful. These positive emotions create fertile ground for joy to flourish, enabling us to savor life's moments and derive pleasure from even the simplest of things.

Positivity also serves as a shield in times of adversity, granting us the resilience to navigate challenges with patience and unwavering strength. A positive attitude equips us to confront setbacks, adversity, and obstacles, propelling us to seek joy even amidst the harshest of circumstances.

Positivity's magnetic effect isn't limited to our internal world. When we radiate positivity, we have a tendency to attract like-minded friendships and favorable circumstances. These positive experiences set in motion a ripple effect, intensifying our joy and perpetuating a cycle of positivity.

It's worth noting that positive emotions, like happiness, gratitude, and love, are not just linked to an improved emotional state but are also associated with reduced stress levels, enhanced immune function, and overall well-being. In fact, maintaining a positive outlook can bolster your immunity.

Moreover, positivity and joy harmonize seamlessly with mindfulness and present-moment awareness. When we cultivate positivity, we become more attuned to the beauty and goodness that envelop us in the present moment. This heightened awareness allows us to immerse ourselves fully in experiences, to revel in the joy they bring, and to deepen our overall sense of well-being.

This ripple effect of positivity and joy extends beyond our individual lives. When we exude joy and positivity, we inspire and uplift those around us. Our positive energy can bring about a transformative influence on others, fostering a sense of connection, spreading happiness, and contributing to the creation of a positive, supportive community. Joy and positivity are entwined in a powerful, transformative relationship that influences multiple facets of our lives.

Embracing positivity is the key to unlocking a life brimming with joy, and it equips us to confront life's challenges with grace and gratitude. Grudges and resentment, when clung to, can be like anchors that contribute to chronic stress and anxiety. Cancer, in itself, presents an overwhelming amount of stress and tribulation. So, consider this your sign to embark on a journey of forgiveness and a more positive life chapter. It's time to forgive and move forward.

Forgiveness offers a lifeline in alleviating these stressors by fostering a profound sense of inner peace and tranquility. Letting go of the pain entwined with hurtful experiences can lead to a substantial reduction in stress levels and an overall enhancement of emotional well-being.

The positive impact of forgiveness extends to our psychological well-being and can reduce symptoms of depression, anxiety, and anger while simultaneously promoting greater self-esteem and self-worth. Through the act of forgiveness, you liberate yourself from the clutches of negative thoughts and emotions that may be hindering your path to joy and happiness.

In the realm of relationships, forgiveness is a potent tool for fostering healthier and more fulfilling connections. It provides the opportunity to transcend the pain and rebuild trust, thus paving the way for deeper and more meaningful bonds. I always like to say that forgiveness opens up a space for more happiness in your life.

When you forgive others, you simultaneously nurture a compassionate attitude toward yourself, which, in turn, improves the quality of all your relationships and allows more joy to flow into your life. The journey of forgiveness is, in essence, a powerful act of personal growth and empowerment. It signifies your ability to rise above the pain and take charge of your own emotional well-being. By forgiving, you reclaim your power and choose not to let the hurt define your life.

Refuse to let cancer, or any other hurt, define your existence. Instead, embark on a path of personal growth, resilience, and a renewed sense of purpose. On your journey toward forgiveness and healing, it's crucial to recognize and allow yourself to feel the pain, for it's in acknowledging the pain that you can release it. Hand it back to God, and treat yourself with the kindness and compassion that you so rightly deserve. Self-compassion entails acknowledging your pain while embracing a non-judgmental attitude toward yourself. Be patient and gentle as you navigate the healing process.

The act of releasing resentment is life-changing. Opt to let go of the negative emotions and resentment that may have been holding you back and hindering your healing journey post-cancer. In this process, establish your "new normal" and set clear boundaries to safeguard yourself from further harm. Your well-being should be your top priority. Surround yourself with supportive and healthy relationships.

Remember that forgiveness and healing are profoundly personal journeys, and they both take time. Life, in essence, is a marathon, not a sprint. Through prayer and forgiveness, you gift yourself the opportunity to heal, grow, and rediscover inner peace, ultimately leading to the discovery of joy after cancer.

____

____

____

____

____

____

____

____

____

____

____

____

____

____

____

____

____

____

____

____